Pictures of Veterinary Embryology

Clemens Knospe

Copyright © 2013
2nd edition 2015
Prof. Dr. Clemens Knospe

LMU- München
Veterinärstr. 13
80539 München
CKnospe@lmu.de
All rights reserved.

ISBN-10: 1494304546
ISBN-13: 978-1494304546

Preface

It is still true what Hamilton in his famous textbook wrote - 'a sound knowledge of Embryology cannot be obtained solely from a textbook and also not without assuming comparative Embryology'. Therefore more than 180 original pictures of embryos of different species, their different parts and organs are presented here. Together with the Pictures of Veterinary Anatomy and Pictures of Veterinary Histology now the complete Veterinary Morphology is available as Mini-Atlas.

Munich, December 2013/15

CLEMENS KNOSPE

CONTENTS

	Preface	3
1	Progenesis	7
2	Early Development	15
3	Stages	23
4	Skin and Derivatives	72
5	Locomotive Apparatus	77
6	Circulatory System	82
7	Respiratory Apparatus	87
8	Digestive Apparatus	91
9	Urogenital Apparatus	97
10	Nervous System	106

CLEMENS KNOSPE

1 PROGENESIS

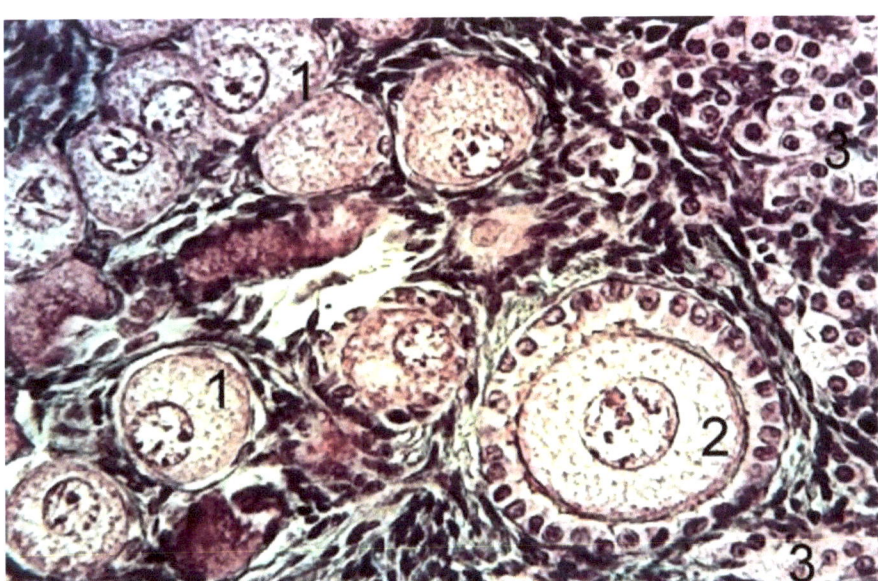

Ovary, cat, GRA, 240x: 1 primordial follicles, 2 primary follicles, 3 intermediate cells.

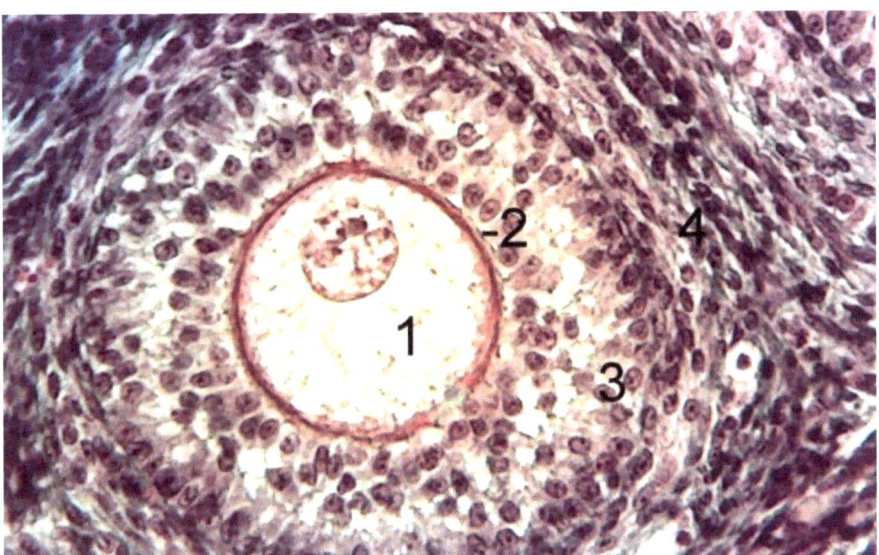

Secondary follicles, Ovar, cat, GRA, 240x: 1 oocyte, 2 zona, 3 follicle epithelium, 4 theca.

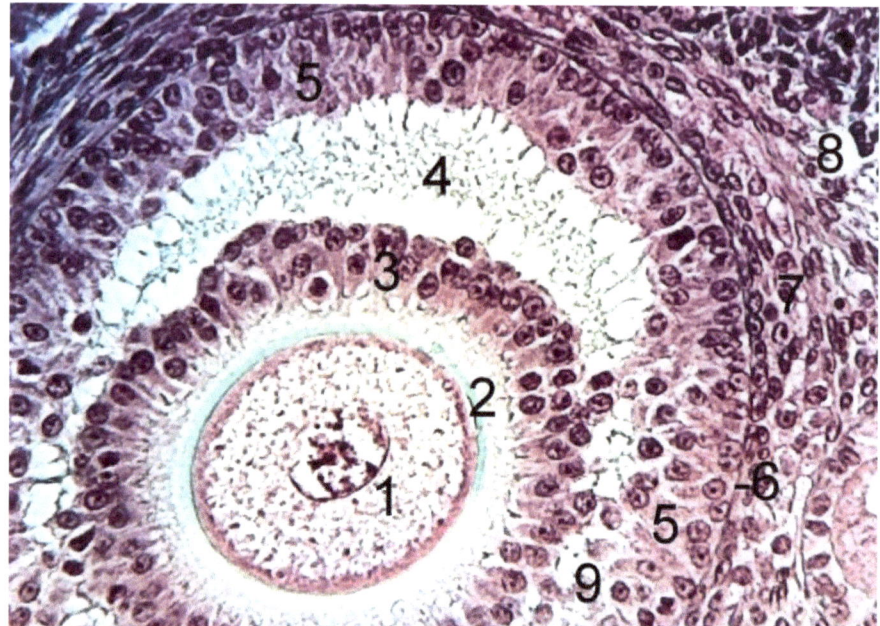

Tertiary follicle, ovary, cat, GRA, 240x: 1 oocyte, 2 zona, 3 corona, 4 antrum, 5 granulosa, 6 basal membrane, 7 internal theca, 8 external theca, 9 cumulus.

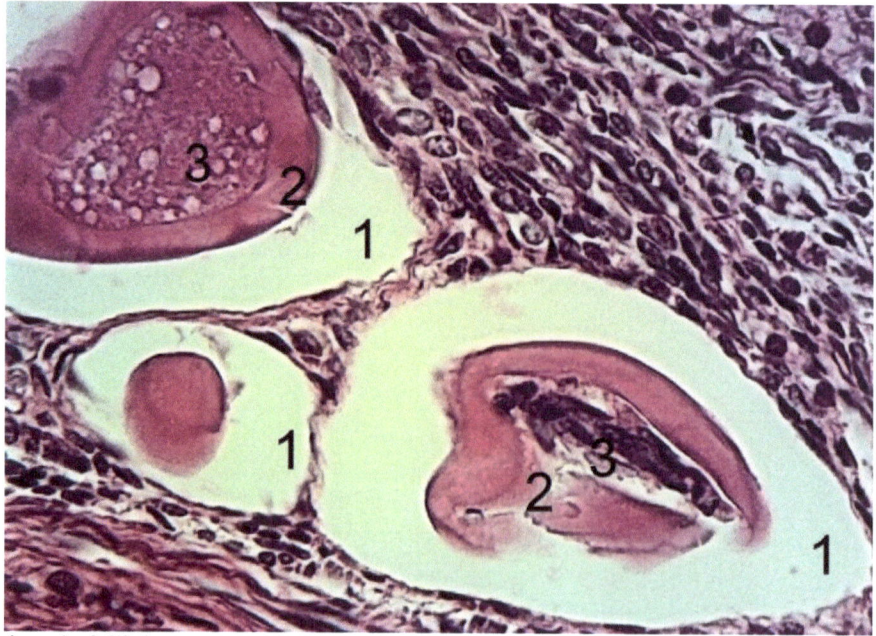

Atretic follicles, ovary, cat, HE, 375x: 1 degenerated follicles, 2 zona, 3 detritus.

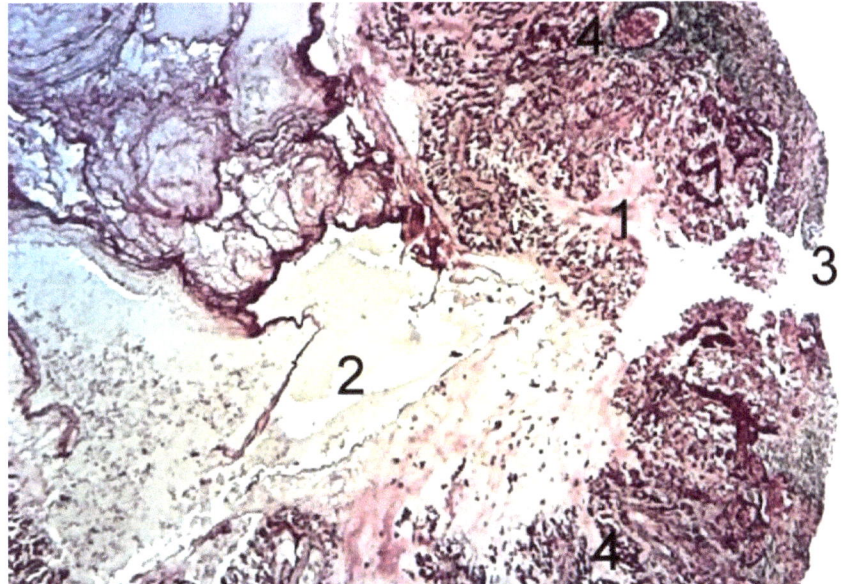

Ovulated follicle, dog, GRA, 25x: 1 luteal body in development, 2 remnants of the follicle cavity, 3 Stigma, 4 proliferating follicle- and theca epithelium.

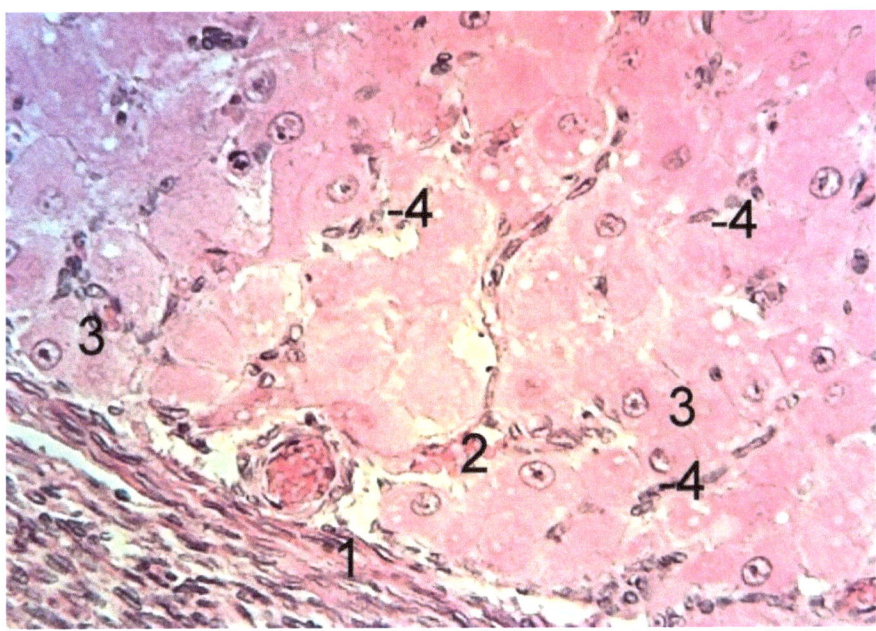

Luteal body, cat, HE, 240x: 1 capsule, 2 capillaries, 3 granulosa luteal cells, 4 theca luteal cells.

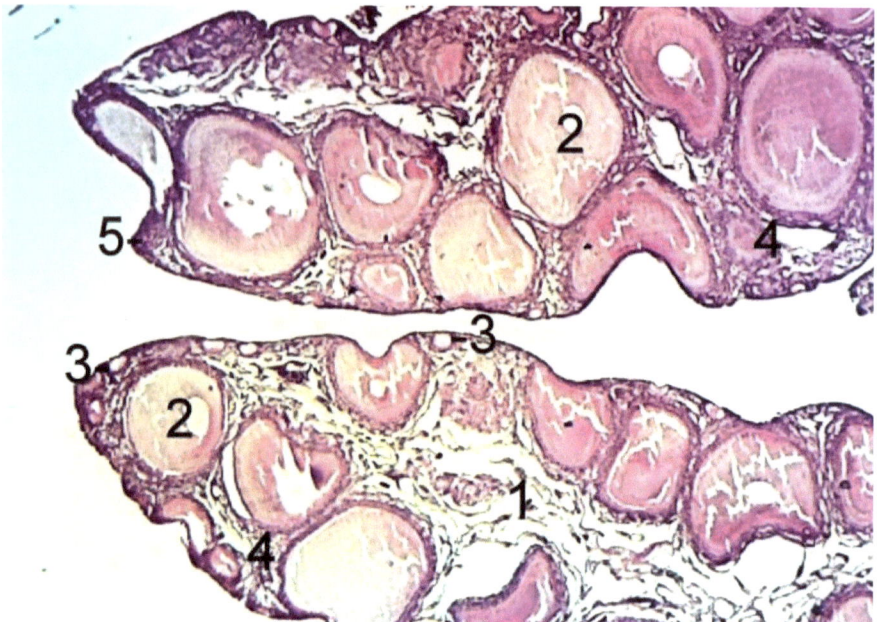

Ovary, chicken, HE, 25x: 1 medulla, 2 tertiary follicles, 3 primary follicles, 4 secundary follicles, 5 peritonel surface.

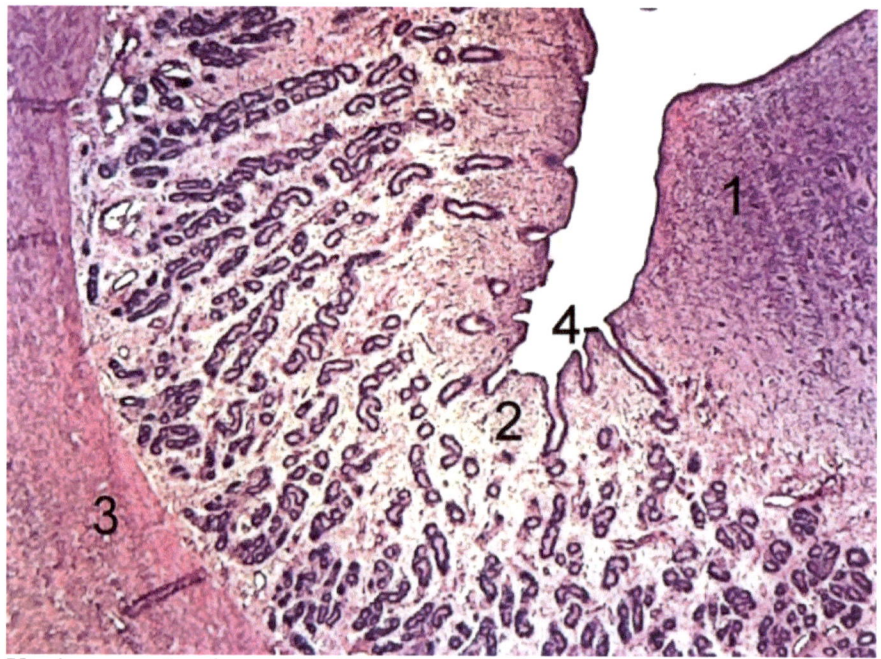

Uterin caruncle, sheep, HE, 25x: 1 caruncle free of glands, 2 uterin glands, 3 myometrium, 4 luminal surface.

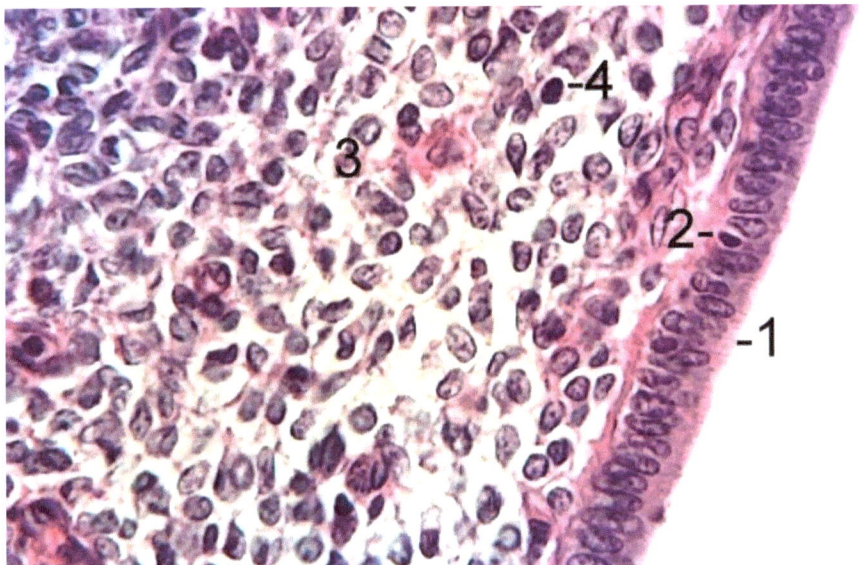

Caruncle, uterus, sheep, HE, 600x: 1 cylindical epithelium, 2 migrating lymphocytes, 3 propria without glands, 4 lymphocytes.

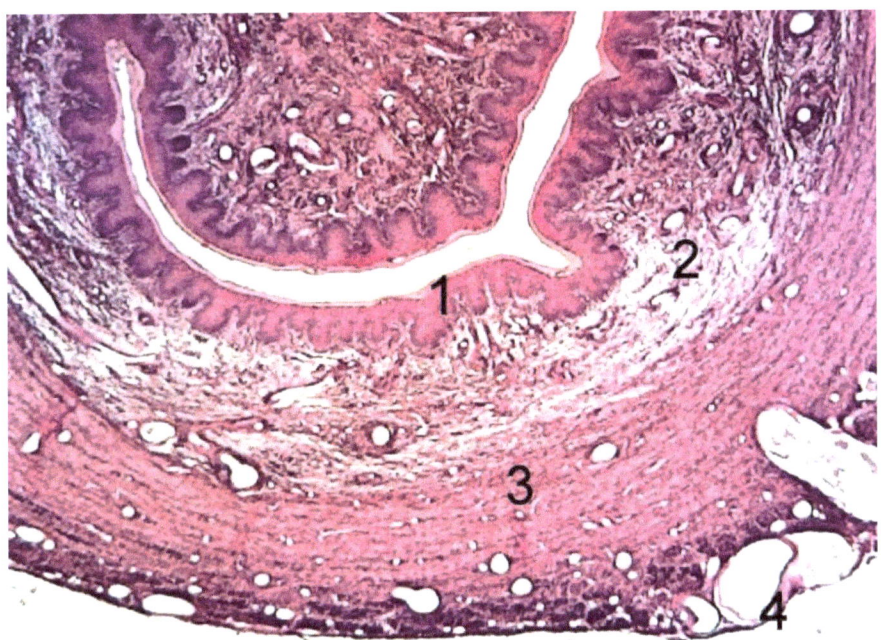

Vagina, cat, HE, 25x: 1 during Oestrus keratinized epithelium, 2 propria, 3 muscle layer, 4 serosa.

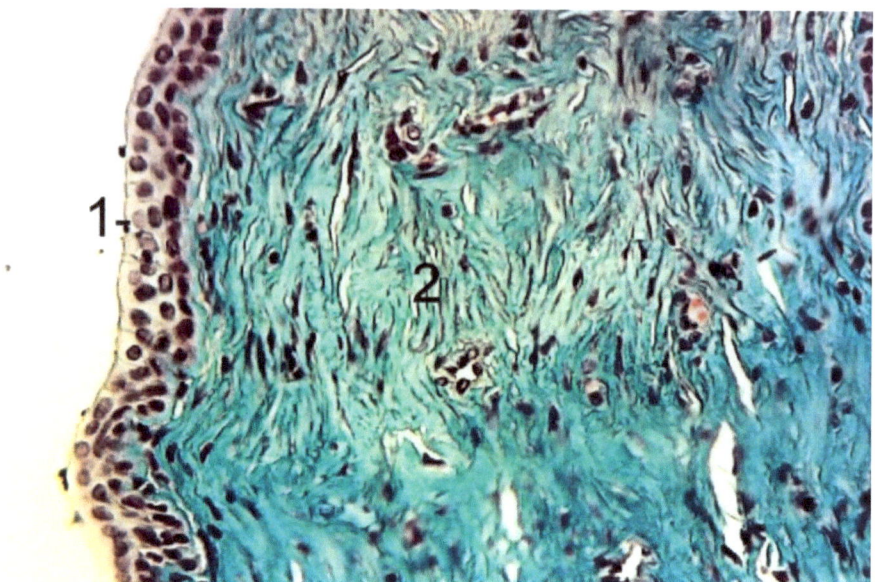

Vaginal epithelium, cat, GRA, 95x: 1 nonkeratinized epithelium during dioestrus, 2 propria.

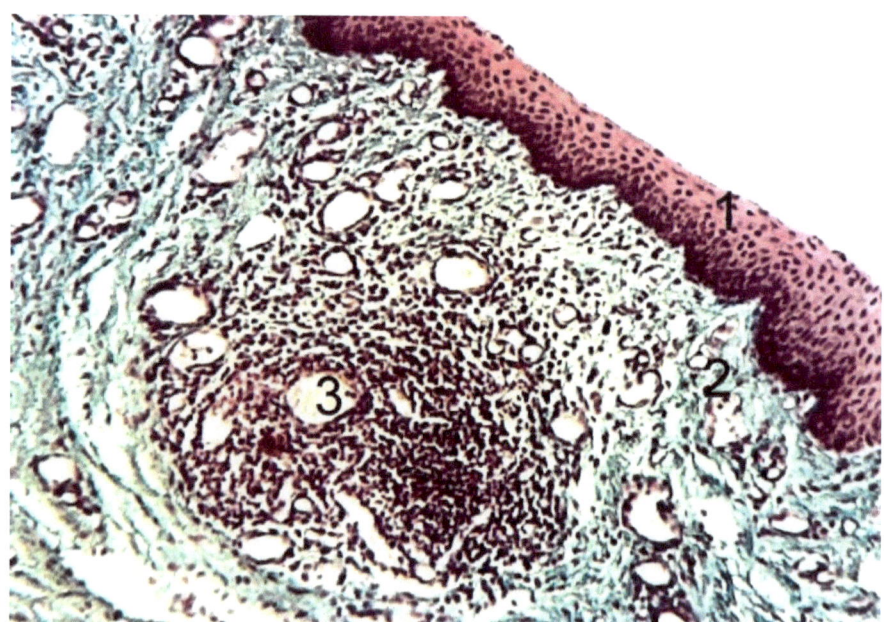

Vaginal vestibulum, pig, GRA, 95x: 1 cutanous mucosa, 2 propria, 3 lymphatic nodules.

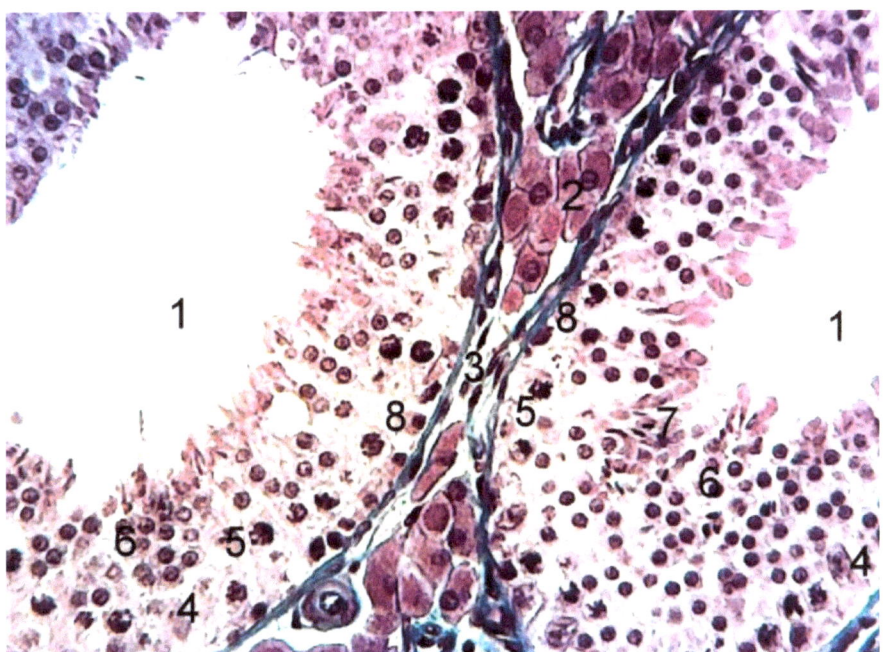

Testis, pig, GRA, 375x: 1 seminiferous tubules, 2 Leydig cells, 3 basal membrane, 4 sertoli cells, 5 Spermatocytes I, 6 spermatids, 7 presperms, 8 spermatogonia.

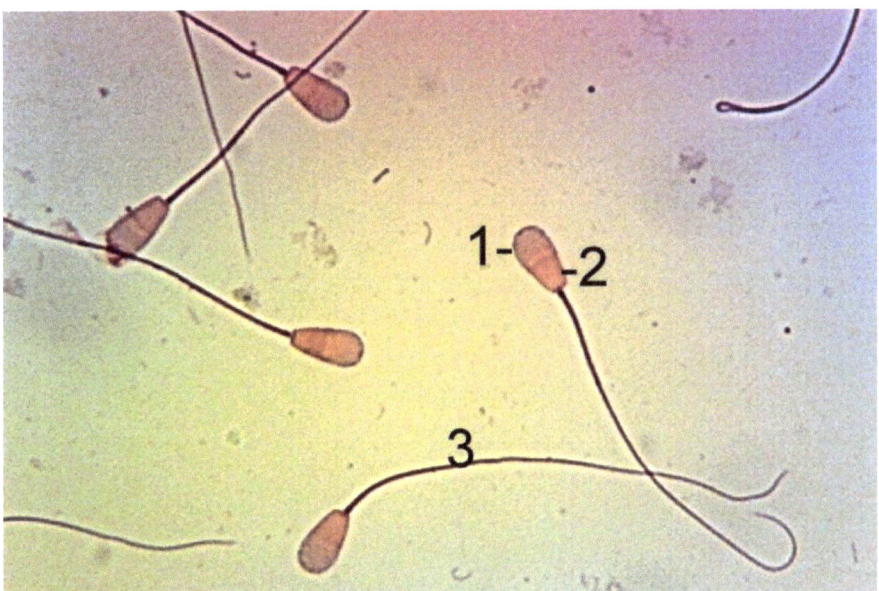

Sperm cells, cattle, Karras, 600x: 1 acrosom, 2 head, 3 tail.

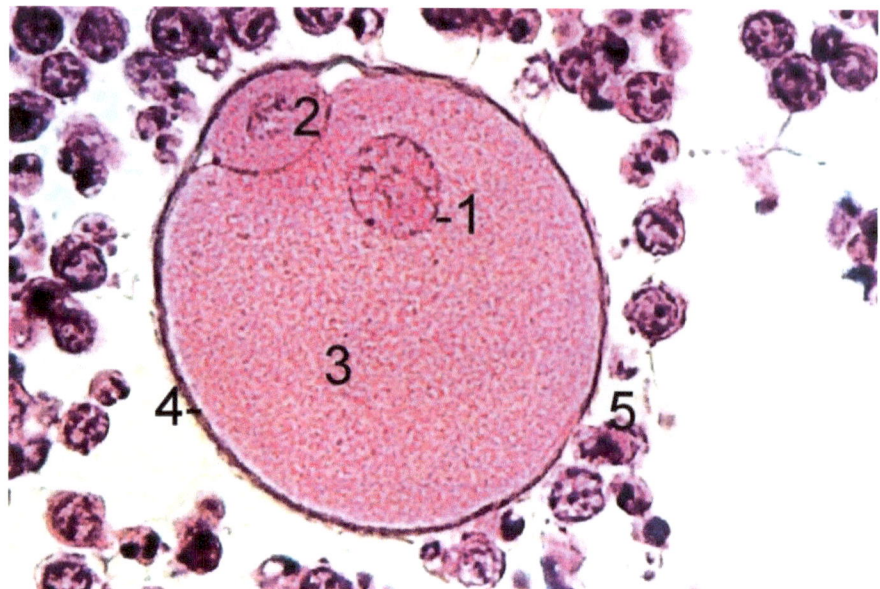

Fertilization, ovum, mouse, 6 hours, cross section, HE, 600x: 1 pronucleus, 2 2nd polar body, 3 cytoplasm of the ovum, 4 oolemm and perivitelline space, 5 remnants of the corona.

2 EARLY DEVELOPMENT

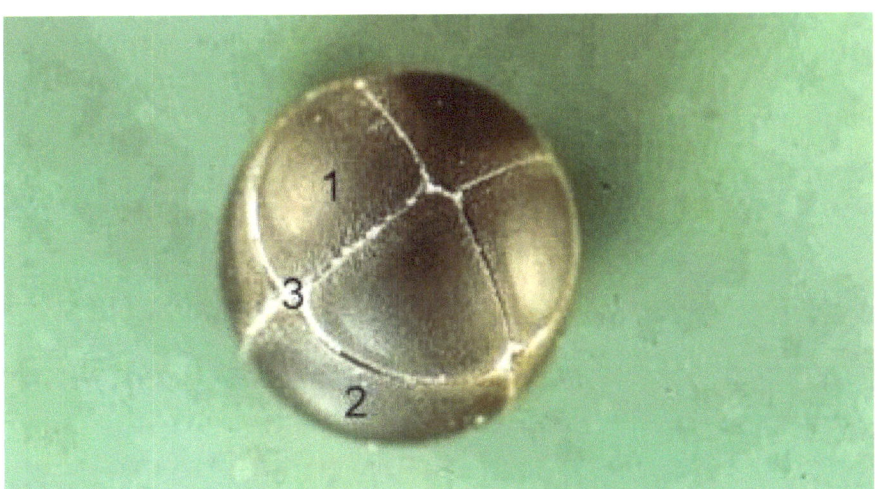

Cleavage, blastumerula (8 cell stage, top), frog, dried, 6x: 1 dorsal micromeres, 2 ventral macromeres, 3 glycoprotein filled clefts.

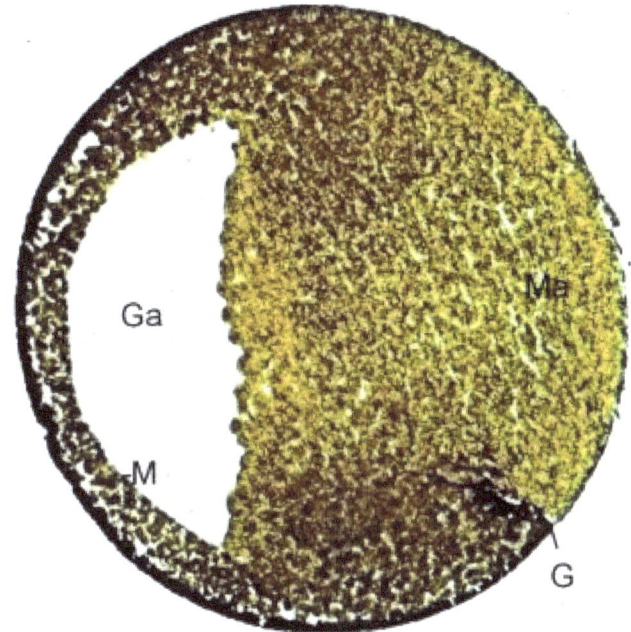

Formation of the germ layers, frog, Pikroblauschwarz, dried, 15x: gastropore (G), gastrocoel (Ga), micromeres (M), macromeres (Ma).

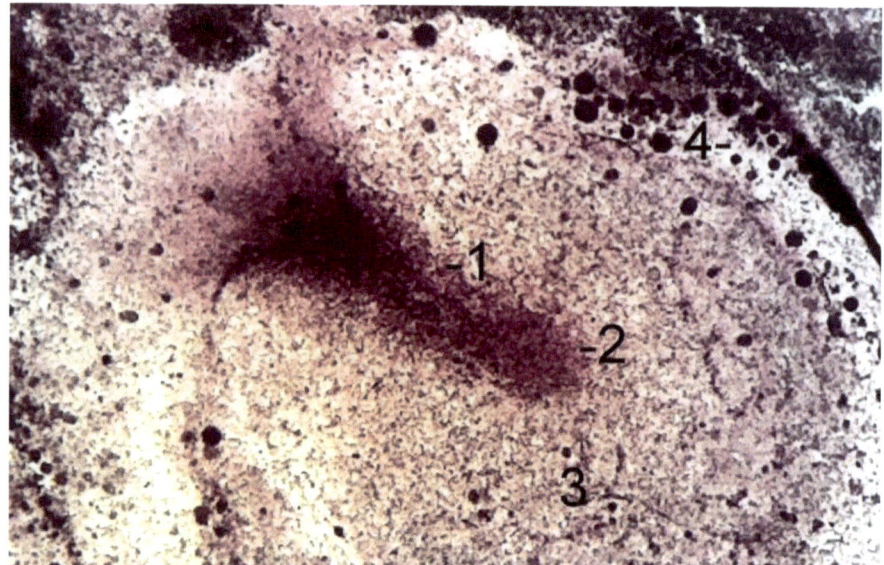

Gastrula, chicken, 10 hours, from top, Carmalaun, 25x: 1 primitive streak, 2 Hensen's node, 3 Area pellucida, 4 Area opaca.

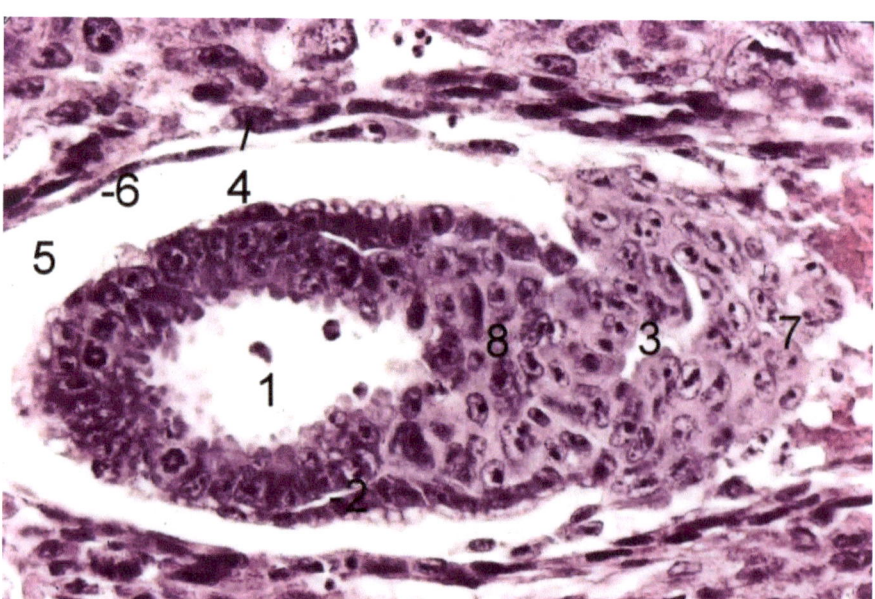

Gastrula, mouse, cross section, HE, 400x: 1 amniotic cavity, 2 coelom, 3 ectoplacentar cavity, 4 ectoderm, 5 yolk sac, 6 entoderm, 7 cytotrophoblast, 8 embryoblast.

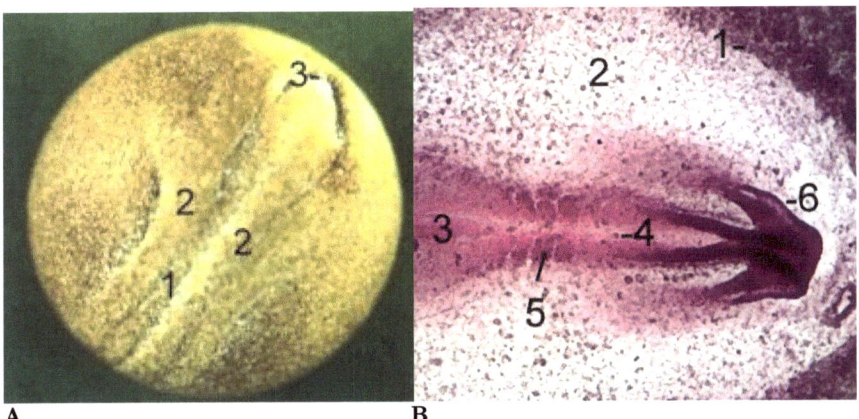

Neurulation, **A** Neurula, frog, from top, dried, 15x: 1 neural groove, 2 neural plate, 3 anterior neuropore; **B** Neurula, chicken, 36 hours, from top, Carmalaun, 25x: 1 Area opaca, 2 Area pellucida, 3 neural plate, 4 neural groove, 5 early somites, 6 head fold.

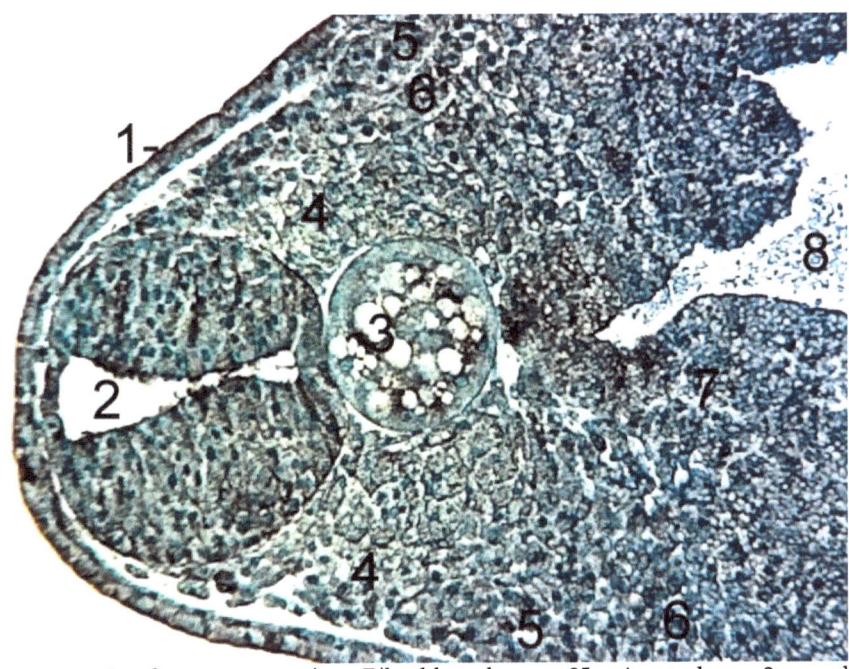

Late neurula, frog, cross section, Pikroblauschwarz, 25x: 1 ectoderm, 2 neural tube, 3 notochord, 4 somite, 5 somatopleura, 6 splanchno(viscero)pleura, 7 entoderm, 8 yolk sac.

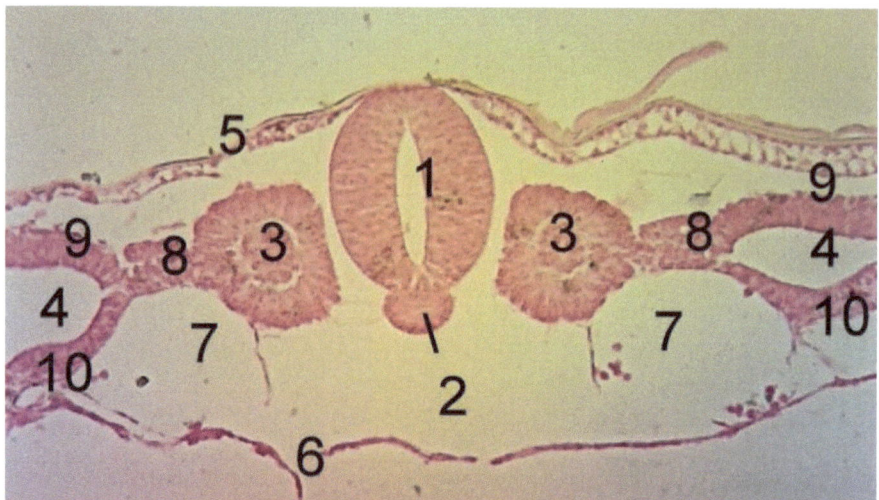

Neurula, chicken, cross section, 36 hours, Carmalaun, 95x: 1 neural tube, 2 notochord, 3 somite, 4 coelom, 5 ectoderm, 6 entoderm, 7 aorta, 8 somite stalk, 9 somatopleura, 10 visceropleura.

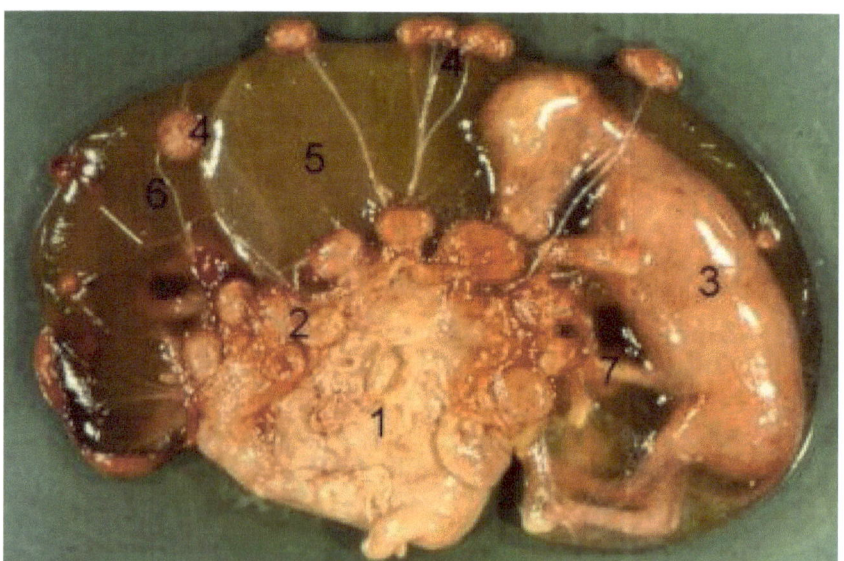

Extraembryonic membranes, cattle, from top: 1 placenta multiplex, 2 cotyledo materna, 3 fetus, 4 cotyledo fetalis, 5 amnion, 6 allantois, 7 umbilical cord.

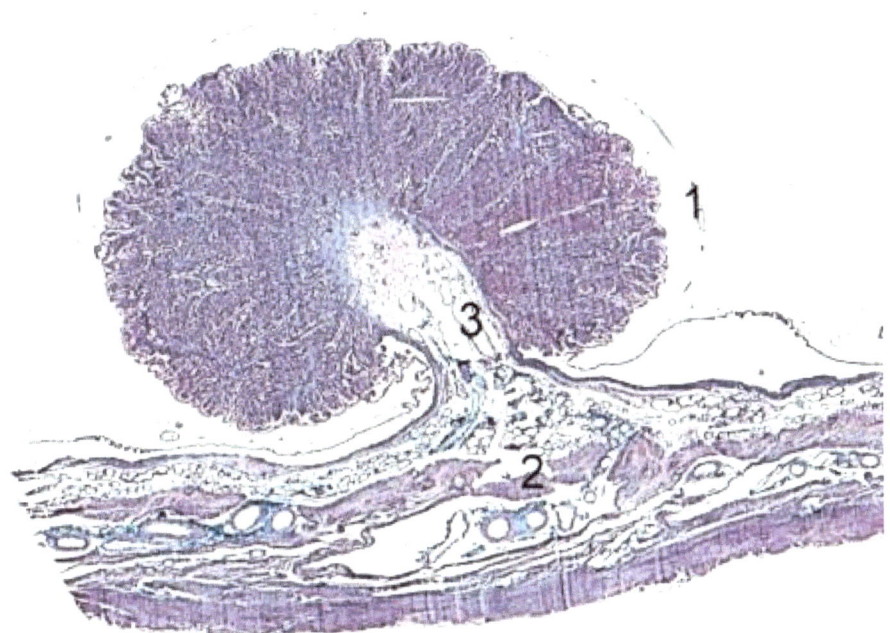

Placentom, cattle, cross section, GRA, 15x: 1 fetal chorion, 2 uterine wall, 3 stalk of the placentom.

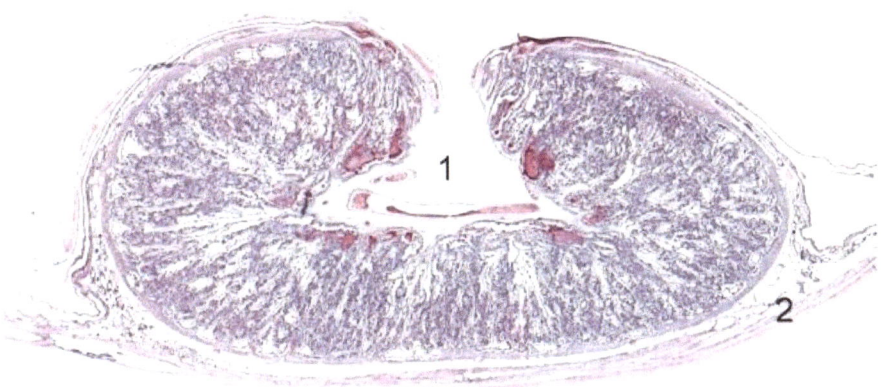

Placentom, sheep, cross section, GRA (Gallocyanin-Chromotrop2R-Anillinblau-trichrom stain), 15x: 1 chorion, 2 uterine wall.

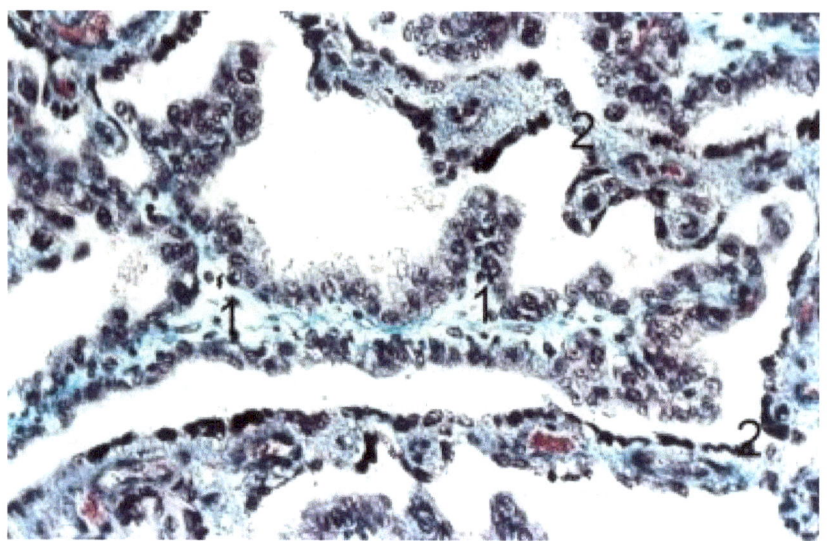

Placentom, sheep, cross section, GRA, 400x: 1 chorionic villi, 2 uterin crypt with symplasma epitheliale maternum.

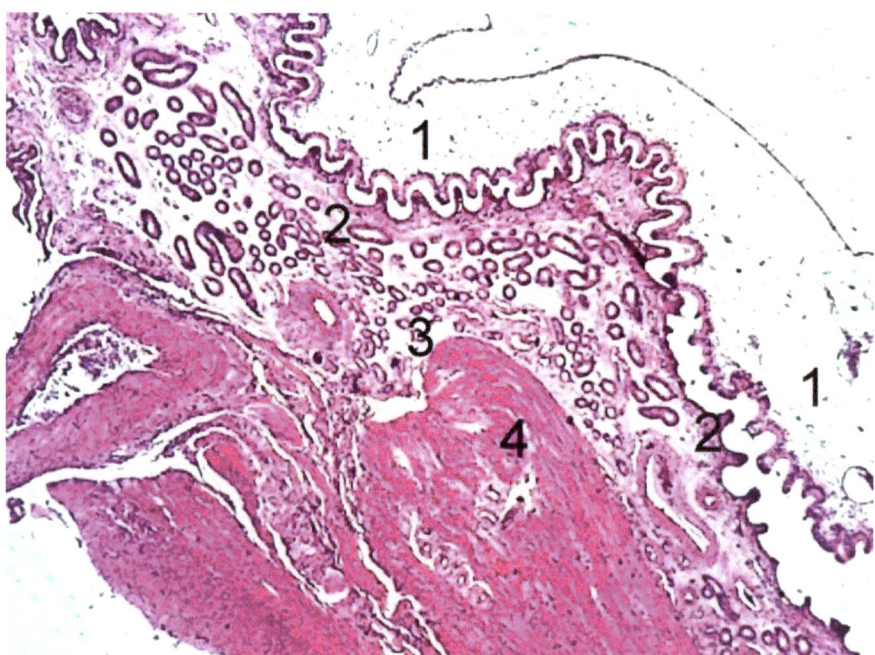

Placenta, pig, cross section, HE, 25x: 1 chorion, 2 uterin mucosa, 3 uterin glands, 4 myometrium.

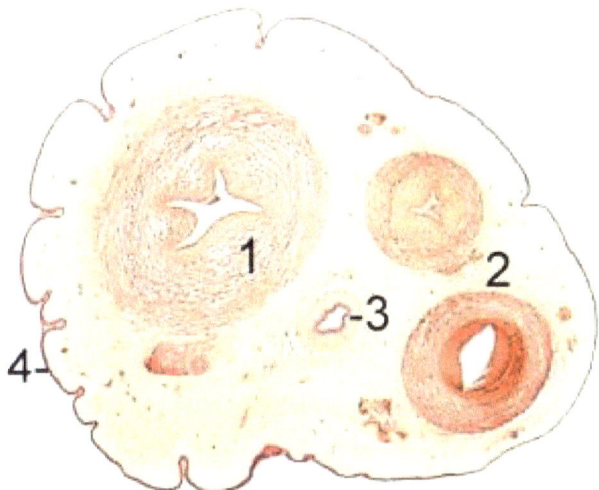

Umbilical cord, pig, cross section, Azan, 25x: 1 umbilical vein, 2 umbilical arteries, 3 urachus, 4 amnion.

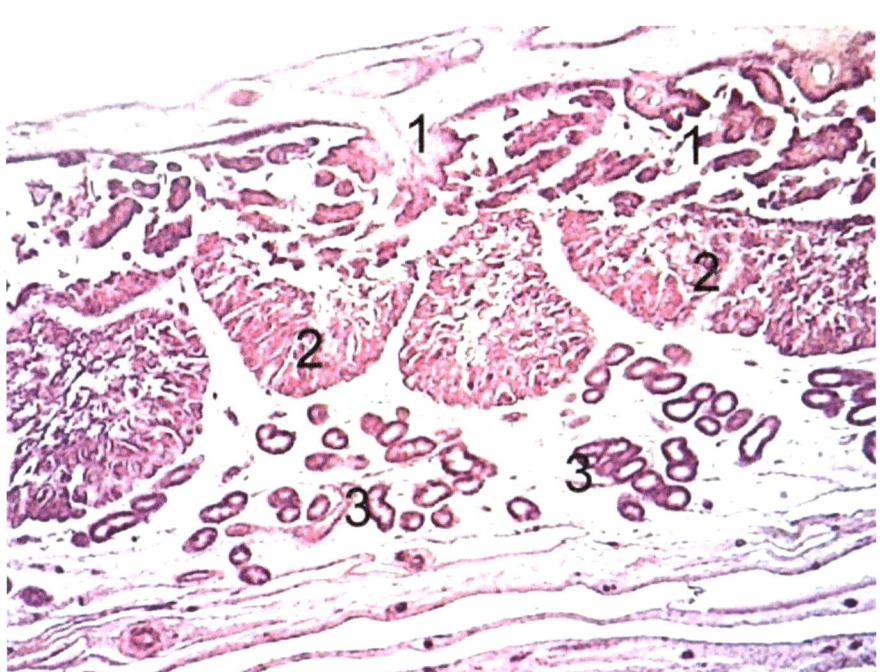

Placenta, horse, cross section, HE, 25x: 1 chorionic villi, 2 uterin mucosa, 3 uterin glands.

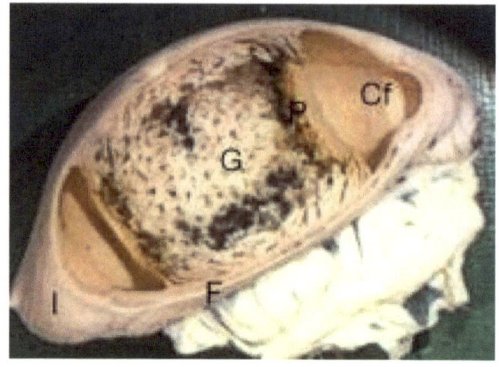

Placenta, cat, uterus chamber opened, half original: chorion leave (Cf), uterus (F), placentar girdle (G), internodium (I), paraplacental region (P);

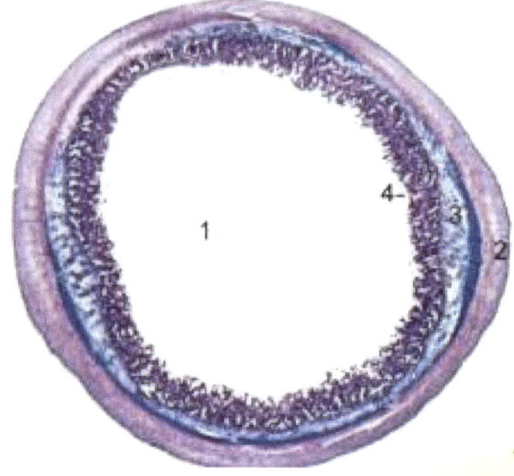

Placentar girdle, cat, cross section, GRA, 15x: 1 lumen of the chamber, 2 uterine wall, 3 endometrium, 4 placenta.

Placenta, cross section, HE, 240x: decidua cells (D) maternal vessels (V), chorionic vessels (F).

3 STAGES

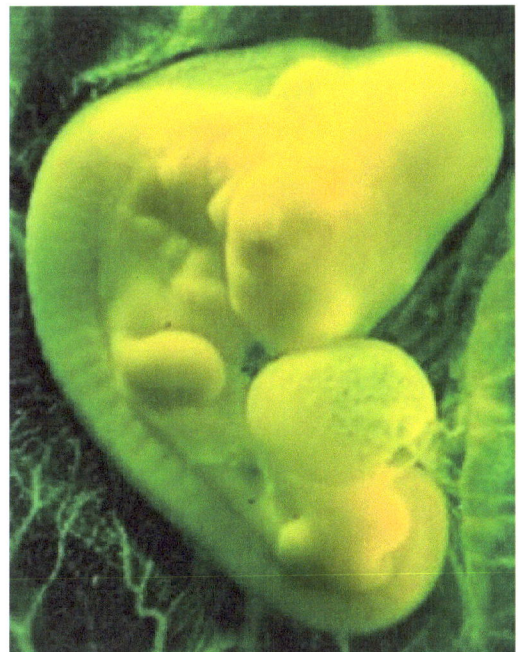

Chicken embryo, 4 days (d) of incubation

Chicken embryo, 4d, longitudinal section, GRA, 15x: 1 midbrain vesicle, 2 heart, 3 mesonephros, 4 intestines.

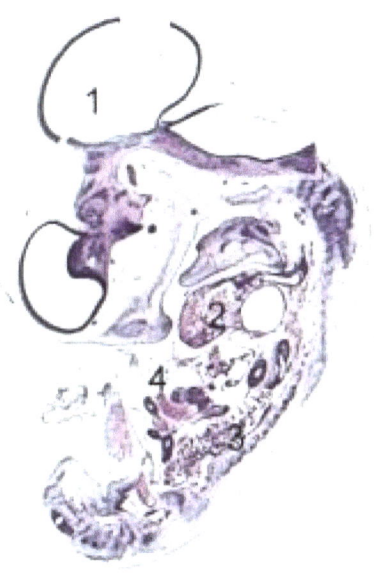

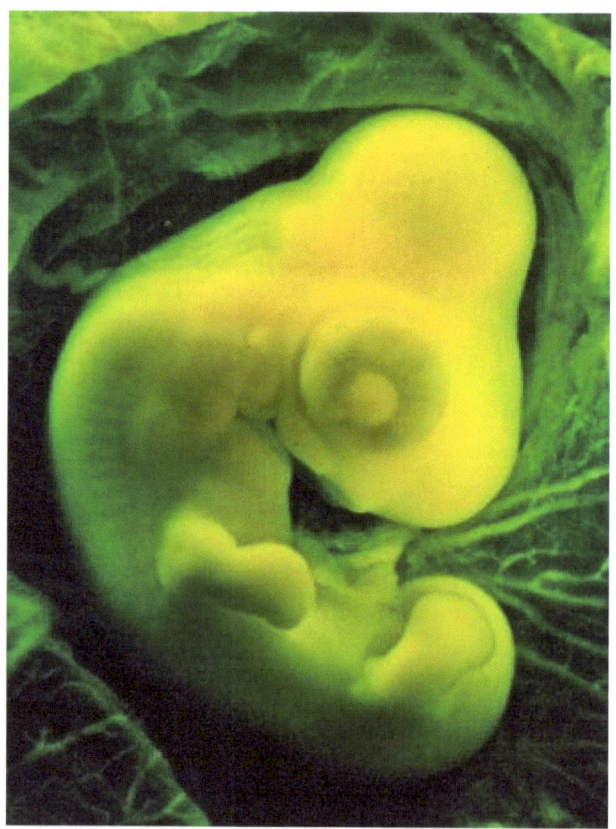

Chicken embryo 5d

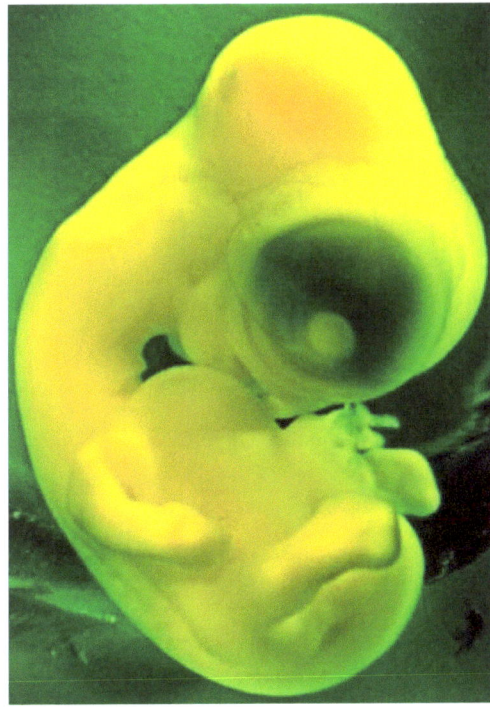

Chicken embryo 6d

Chicken embryo, 6d, longitudinal, HE, 15x: 1 midbrain vesicle, 2 heart, 3 liver, 4 gizzard, 5 lung.

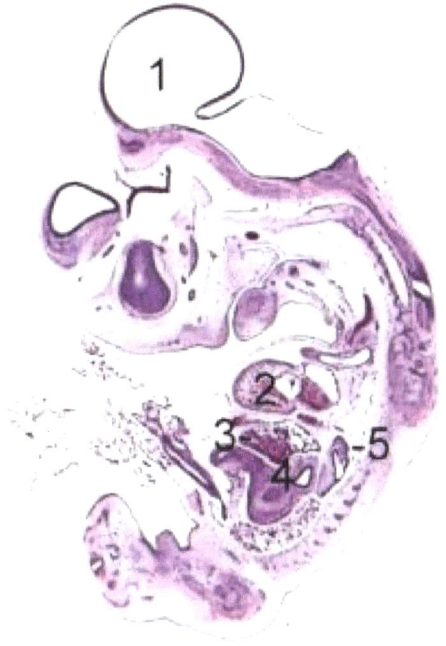

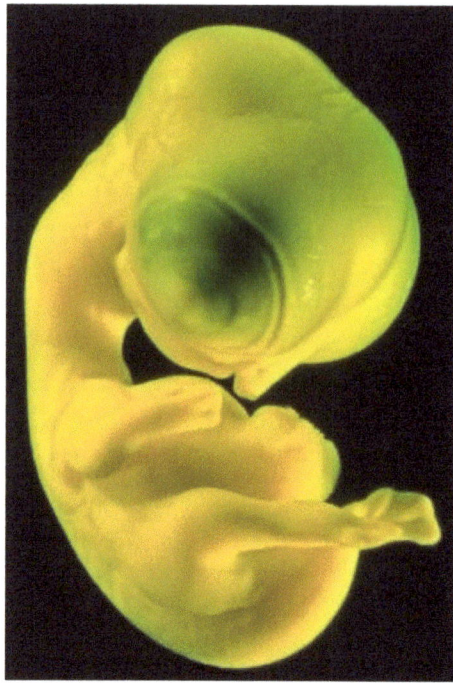

Chicken embryo 7d

Chicken embryo, 7d, longitudinal, HE, 15x: 1 forebrain vesicle, 2 inner ear, 3 spinal cord, 4 heart, 5 lung, 6 stomach, 7 gizzard, 8 intestines.

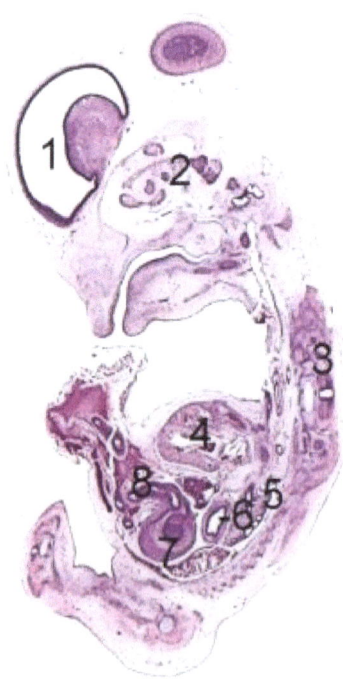

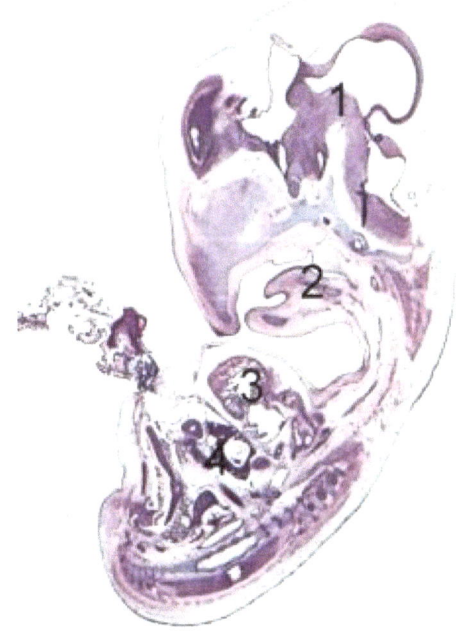

Chicken embryo, 9d, longitudinal, GRA, 15x: 1 midbrain, 2 tongue, 3 heart, 4 gizzard.

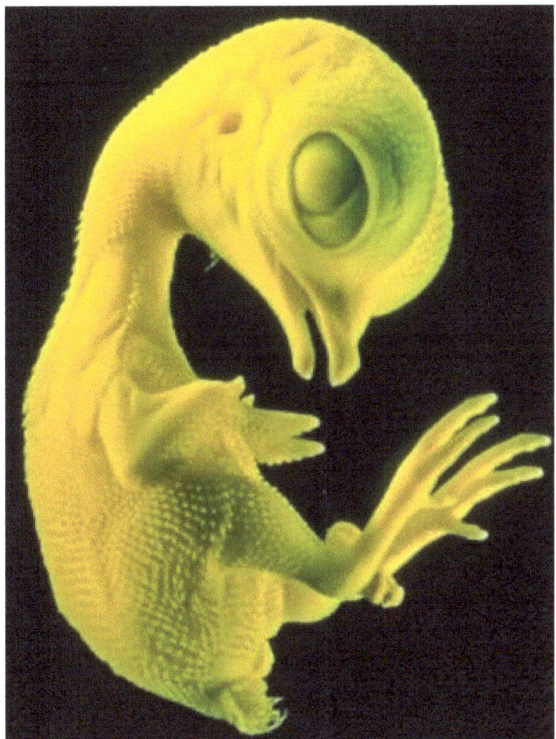

Chicken embryo 10d

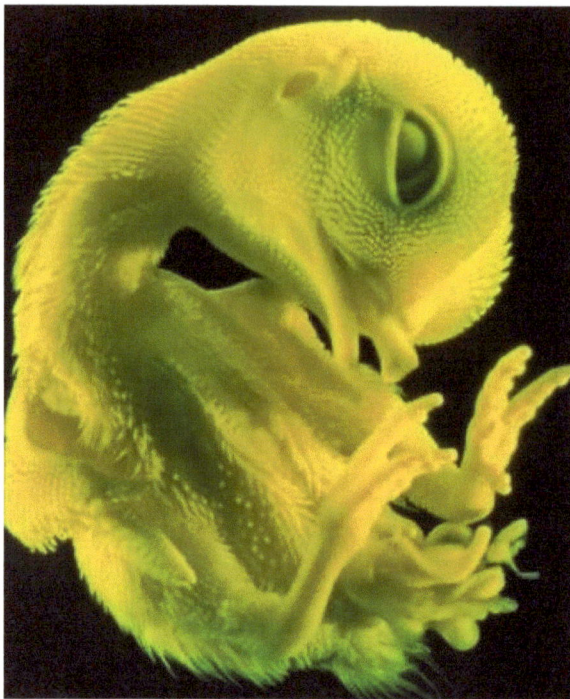

Chicken embryo 11d

Chicken embryo 11d, longitudinal, GRA, 15x: 1 midbrain, 2 heart, 3 gizzard, 4 spinal cord and vertebral column, 5 kidney.

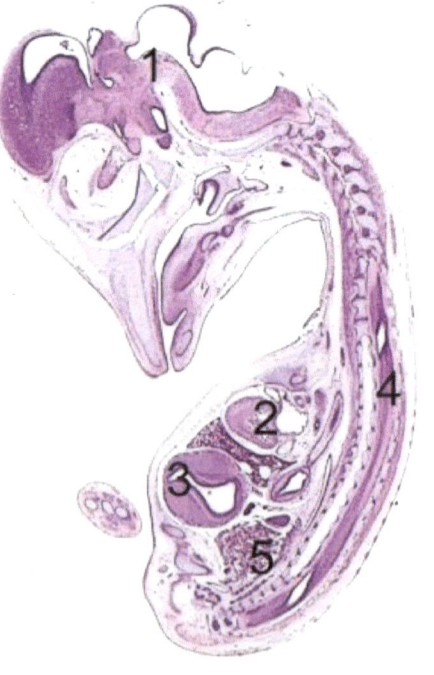

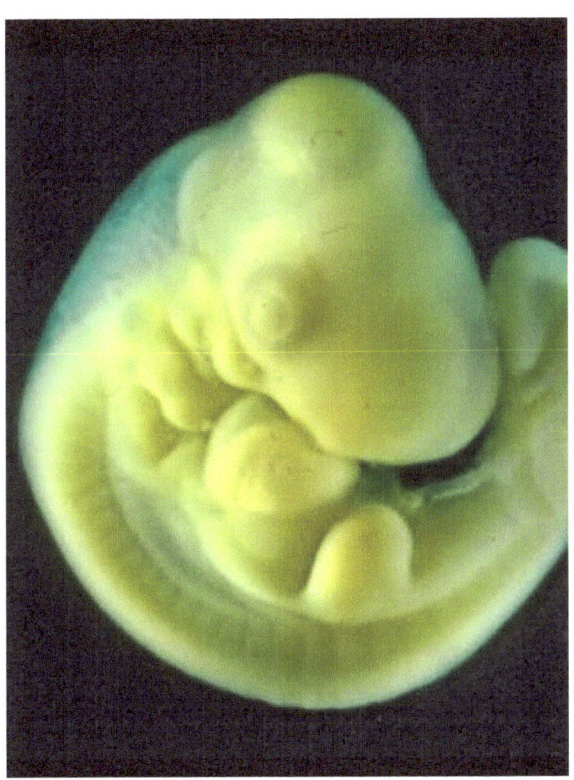

Duck embryo 5d

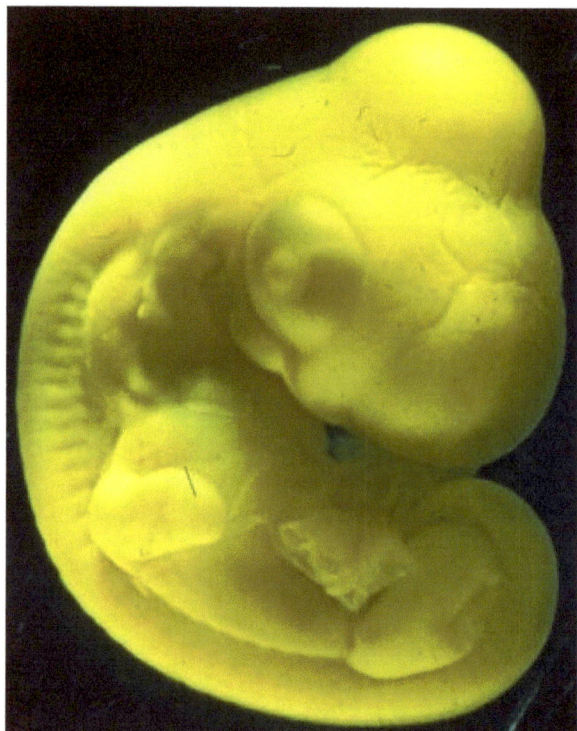

Duck embryo 6d

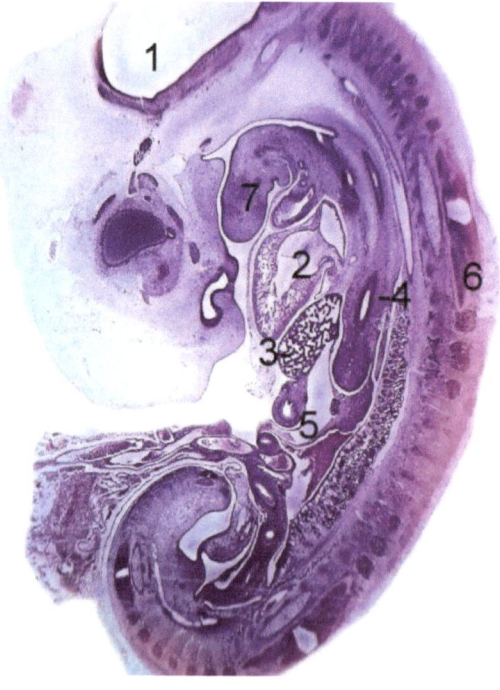

Duck embryo, 6d, longitudinal, HE, 15x: 1 hindbrain, 2 heart, 3 liver, 4 lung, 5 intestines, 6 spinal cord, 7 mandibular process of the first pharyngeal arch.

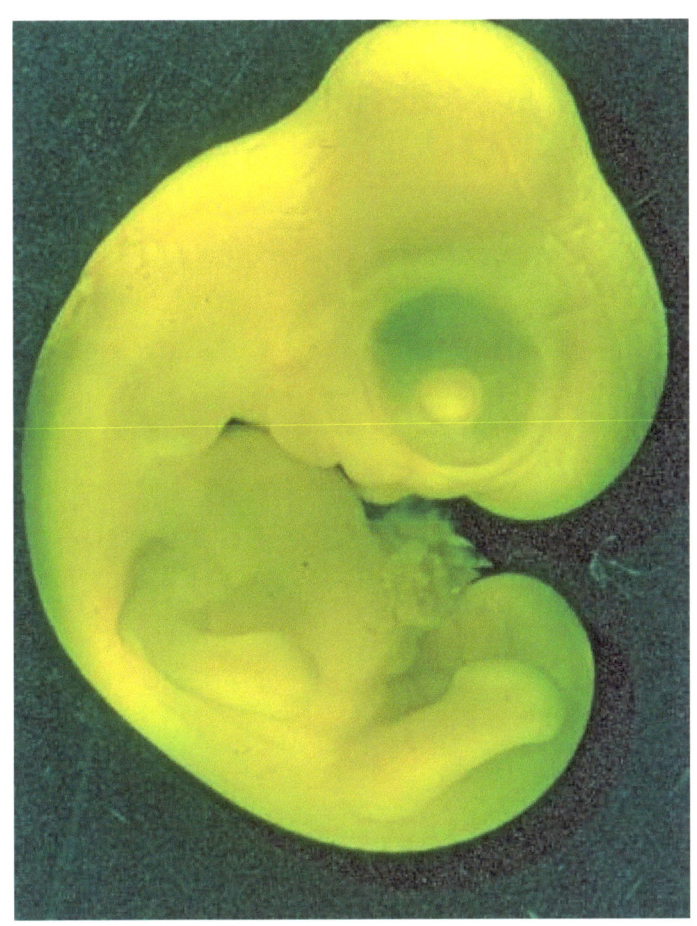

Duck embryo 7d

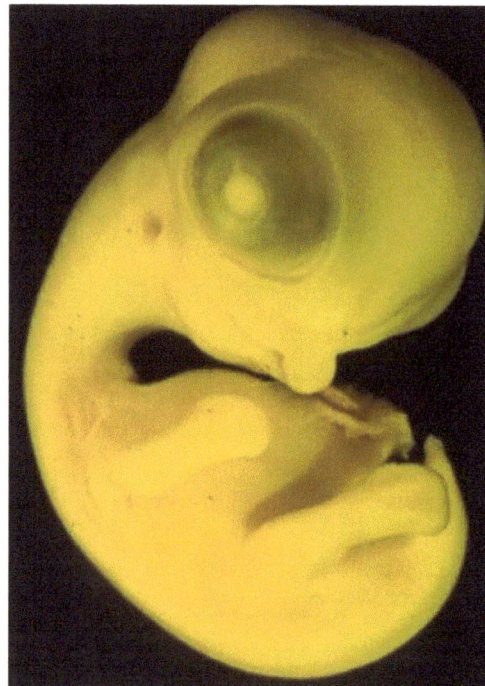

Duck embryo 8d

Duck embryo, 8d, longitudinal section, GRA 15x: 1 forebrain vesicle, 2 neural tube, 3 heart, 4 gizzard, 5 liver.

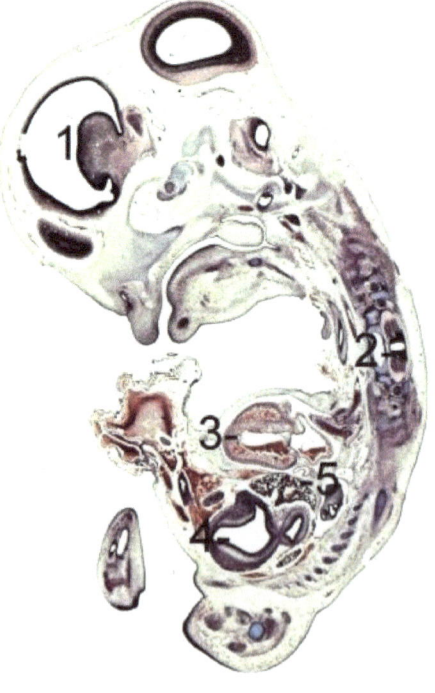

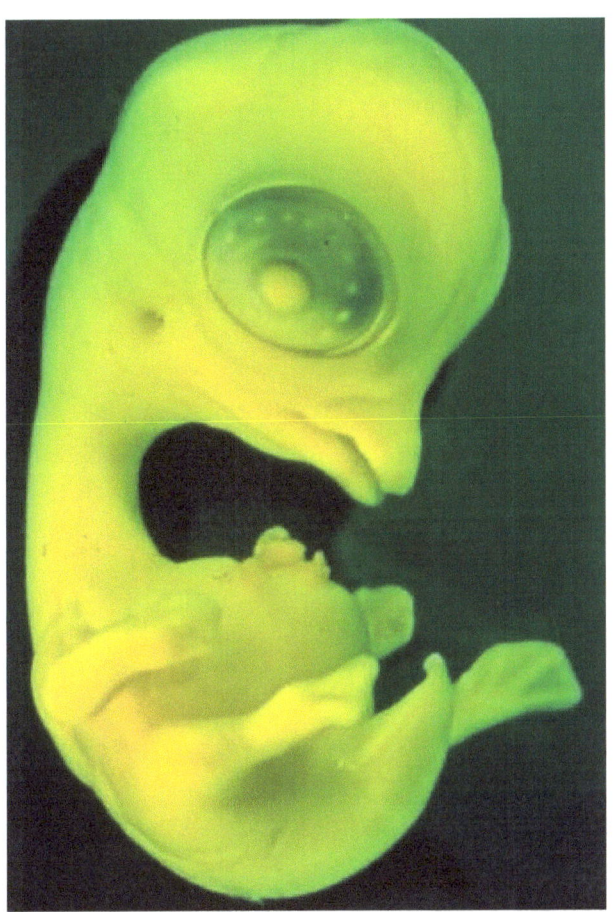

Duck embryo 10d

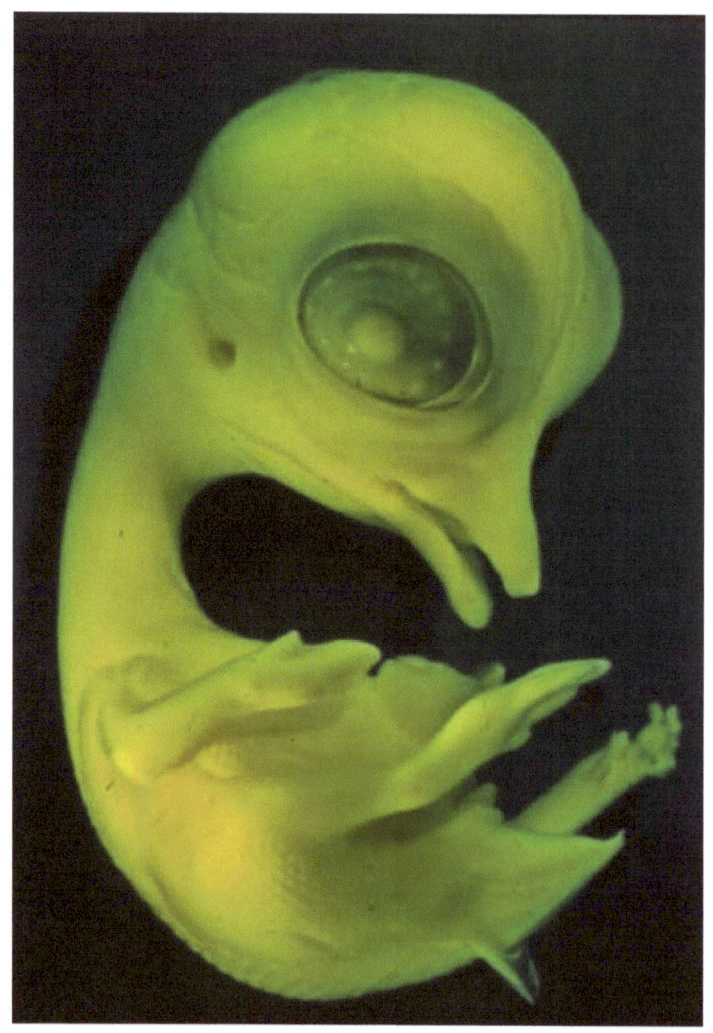

Duck embryo 11d

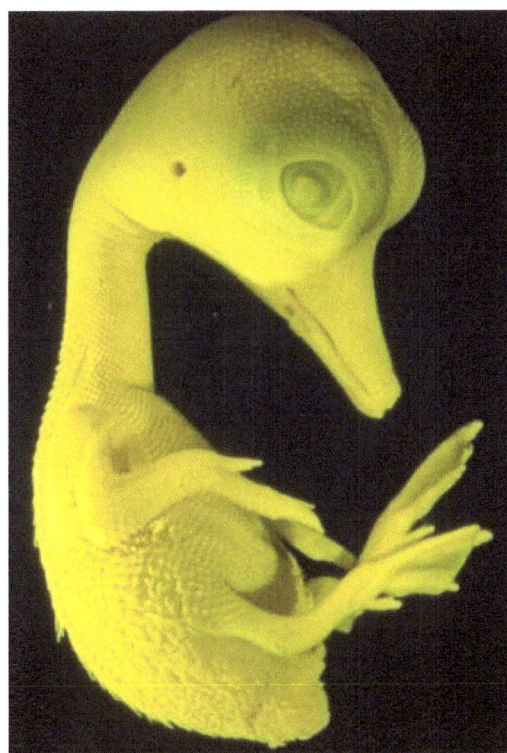

Duck embryo 13d

Duck embryo, 13d, longitudinal, HE, 15x: 1 midbrain, 2 eye, 3 vertebral column, 4 shoulder girdle, 5 liver, 6 heart, 7 hindlimb.

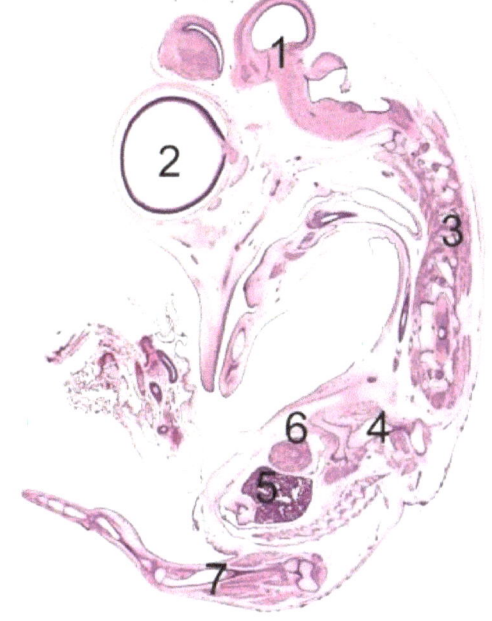

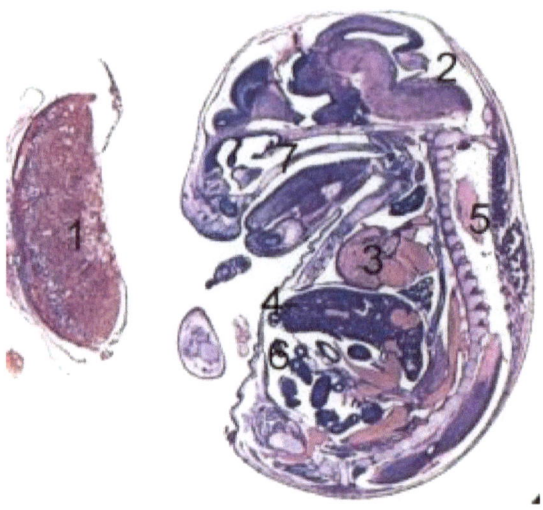

Mouse embryo, prenatal, HE, 15x: 1 placenta, 2 hindbrain, 3 heart, 4 liver, 5 vertebral column and spinal cord, 6 intestines, 7 pharynx.

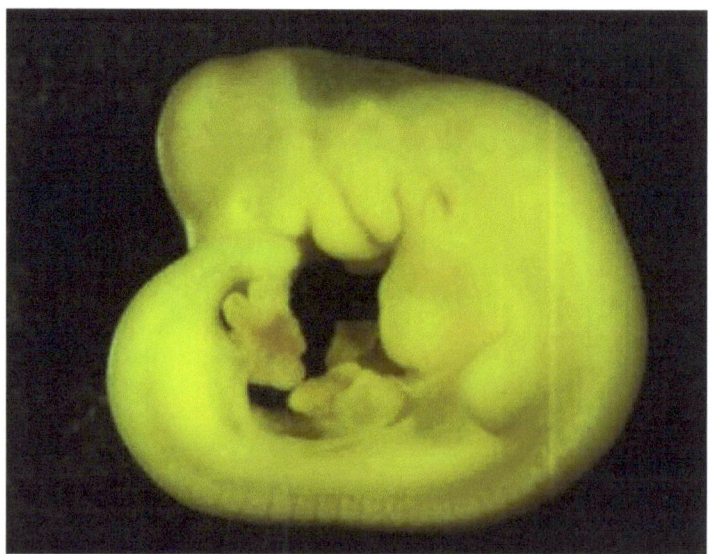

Cat embryo 17d

Pictures of Veterinary Embryology

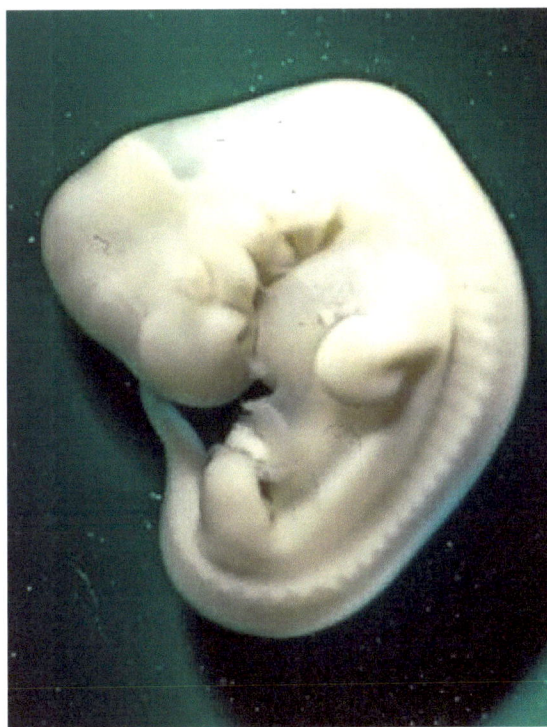

Cat embryo 20d

Cat embryo, 20 days, longitudinal section, HE, 15x: 1 rhombencephalon, 2 heart, 3 lung, 4 liver, 5 stomach.

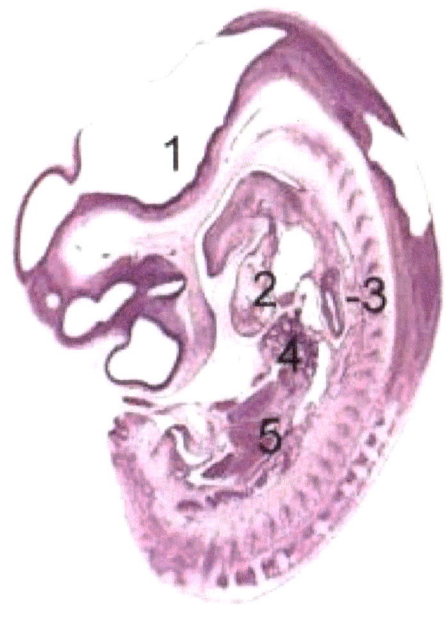

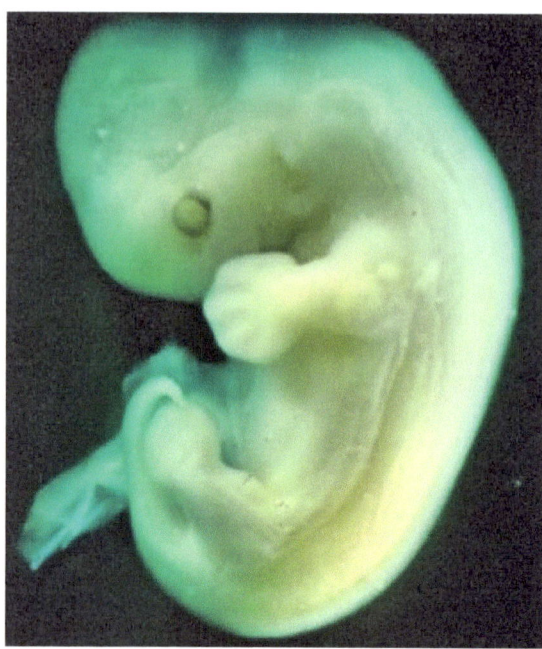

Cat embryo 22d

Cat embryo, 22 days, longitudinal section, HE, 15x: 1 rhombencephalon, 2 heart, 3 neural tube, 4 stomach, 5 liver, 6 mesonephros.

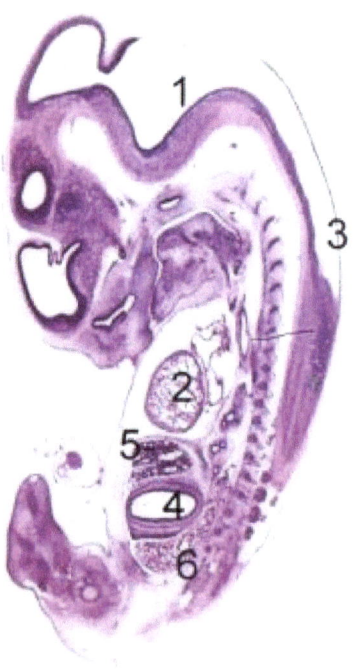

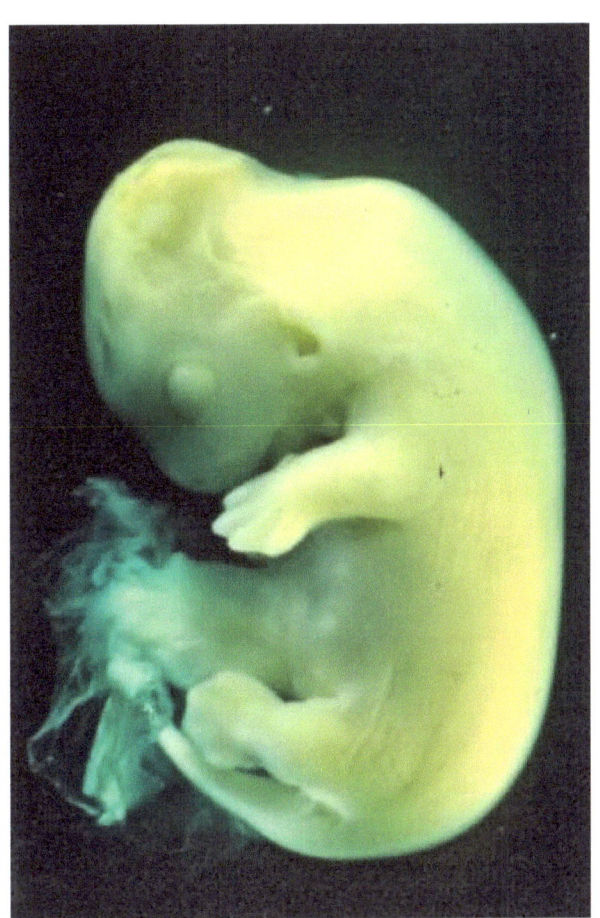

Cat embryo 25d

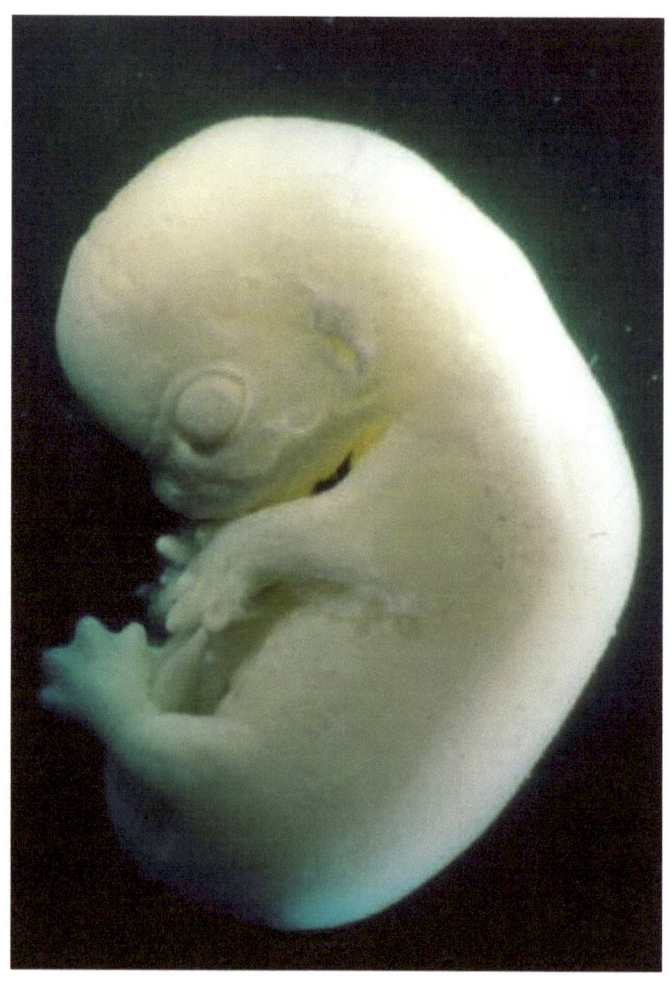

Cat embryo 26d

Pictures of Veterinary Embryology

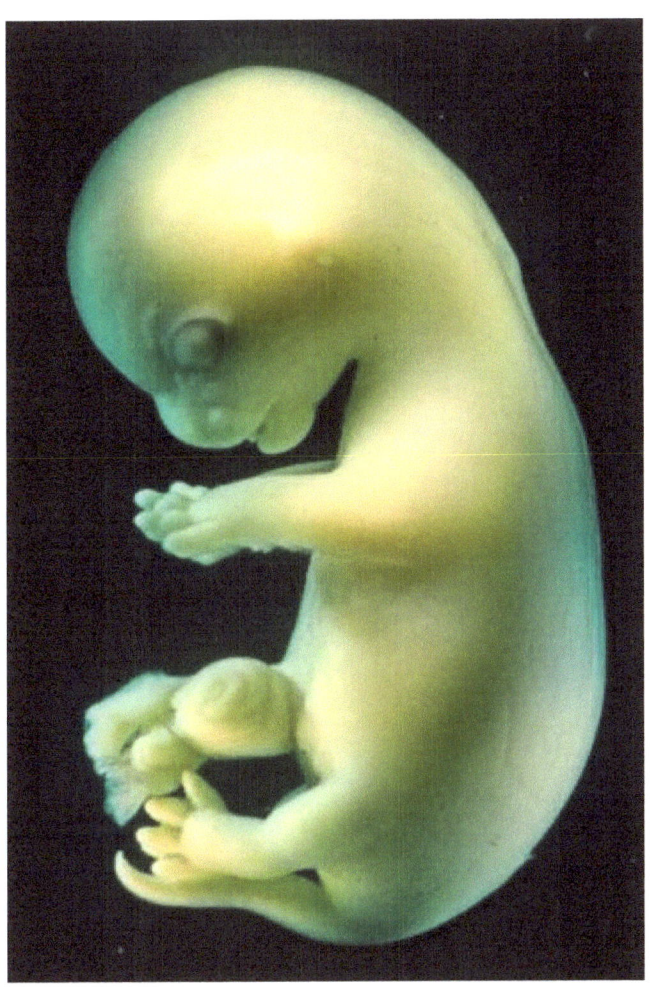

Cat fetus 28d

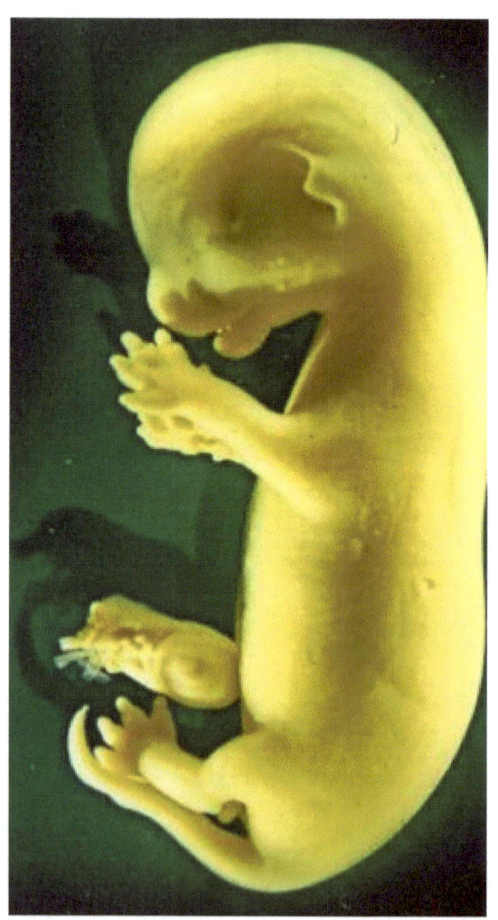

Cat fetus 30d

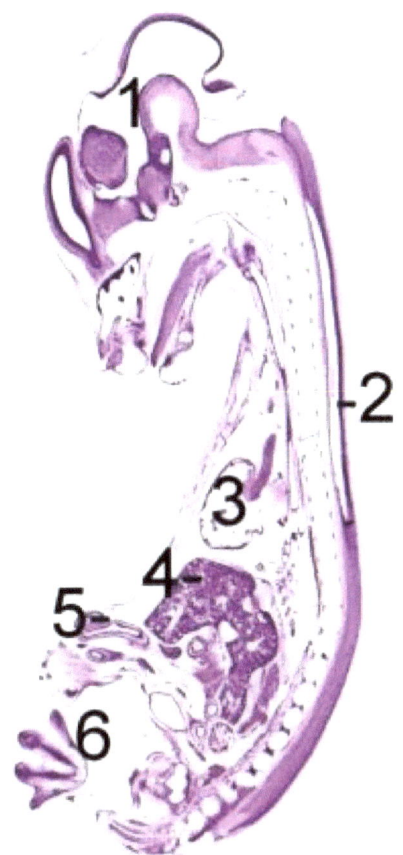

Cat fetus 30 days, longitudinal section, HE, 12x: 1 brain, 2 spinal cord, 3 heart, 4 liver, 5 intestinal herniation, 6 limb bud.

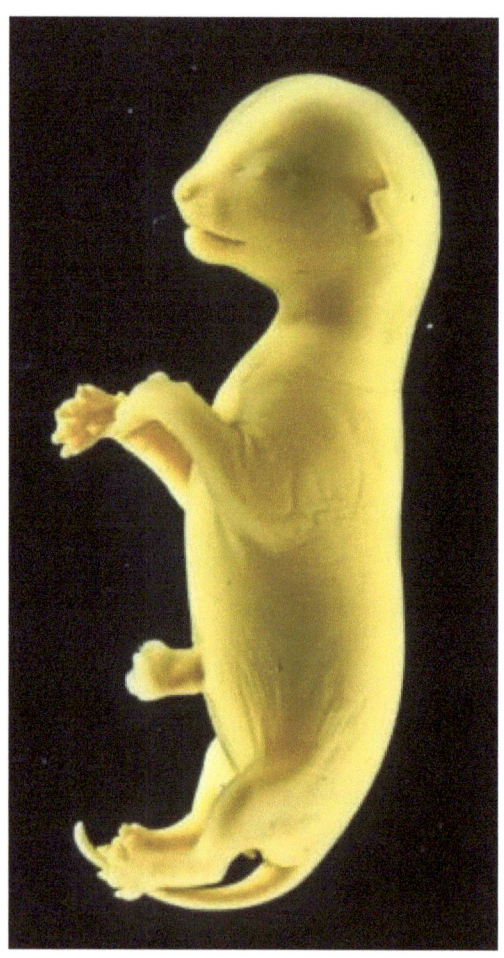

Cat fetus 32d

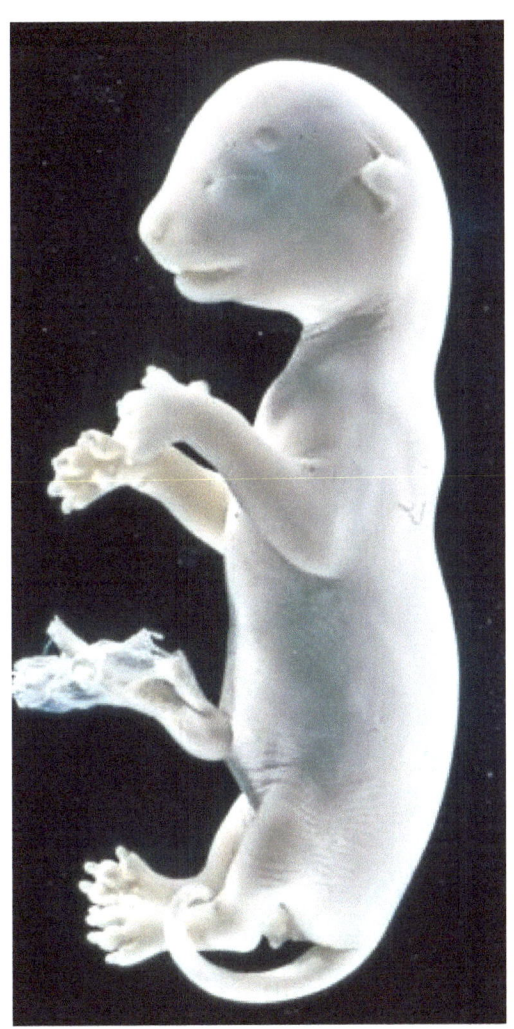

Cat fetus 38d

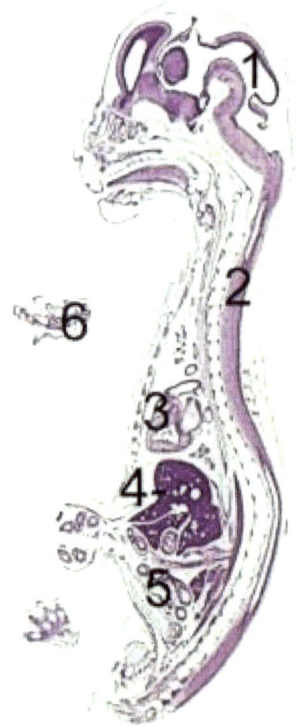

Cat fetus, 38 days, longitudinal section, GRA, 8x: 1 brain, 2 spinal cord and vertebral column, 3 heart, 4 liver, 5 intestines, 6 paw.

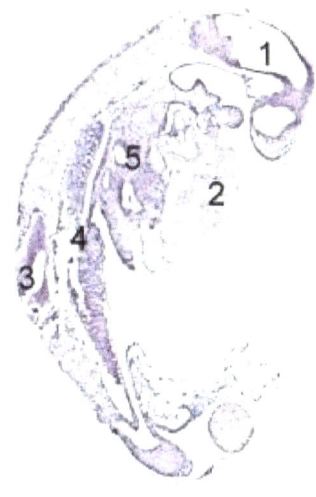

Sheep embryo 6 mm CRL (Crown-Rump-Length), longitudinal section, HE: 1 deuterencephalon, 2 heart, 3 neural tube, 4 mesonephros, 5 gut.

Sheep embryo 9 mm CRL, longitudinal section, HE: 1 rhombencephalon, 2 spinal ganglia, 3 heart, 4 liver, 5 mesonephros, 6 intestines.

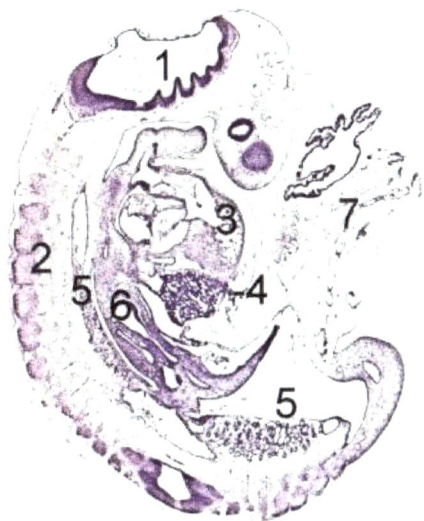

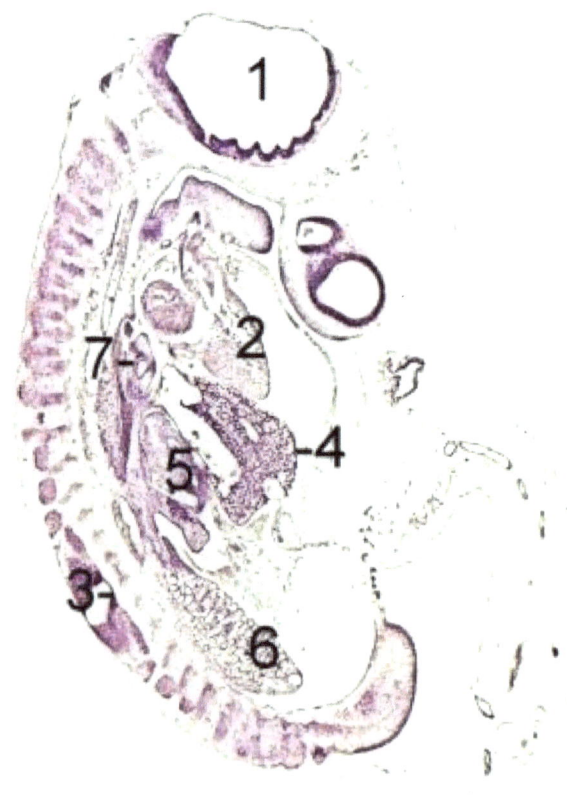

Sheep embryo 9 mm CRL

Sheep embryo 16 mm CRL, longitudinal section, HE: 1 rhomencephalon, 2 heart, 3 neural tube, 4 liver, 5 intestines, 6 mesone-phros.

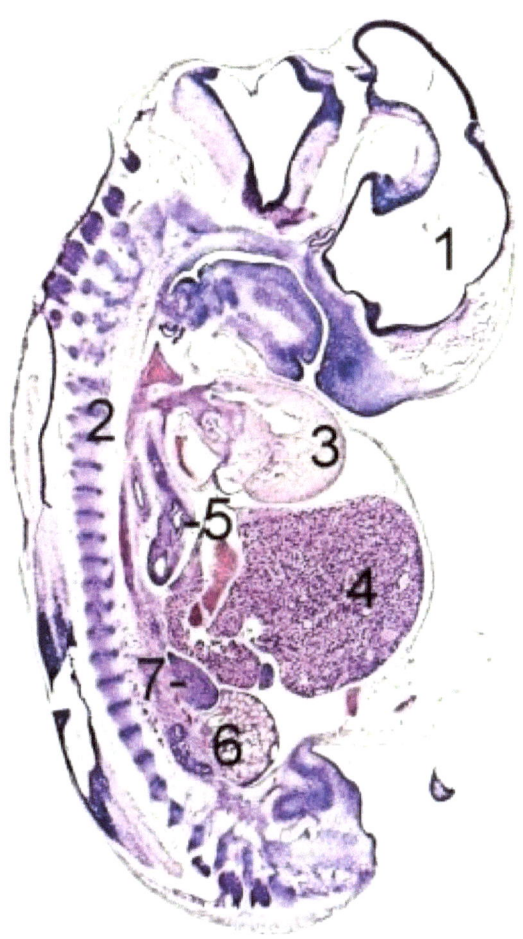

Sheep embryo 19 mm CRL, longitudinal section, HE: 1 forebrain, 2 vertebral column, 3 heart, 4 liver, 5 lung, 6 mesonephros, 7 gonad.

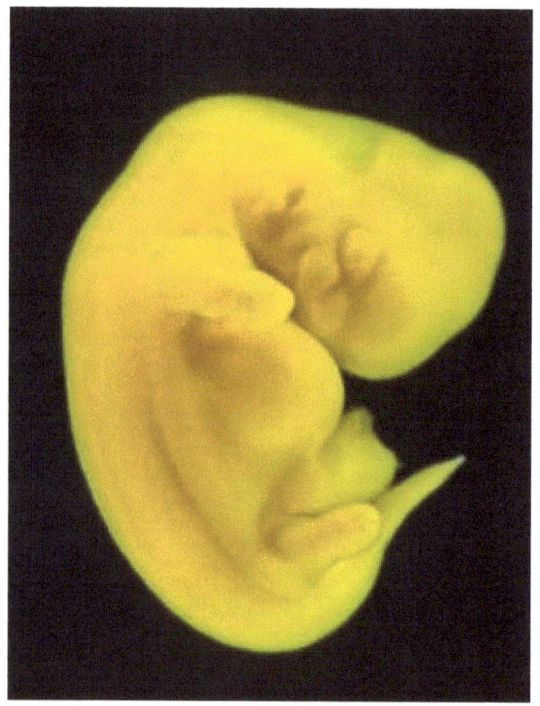

Sheep embryo 25 mm CRL

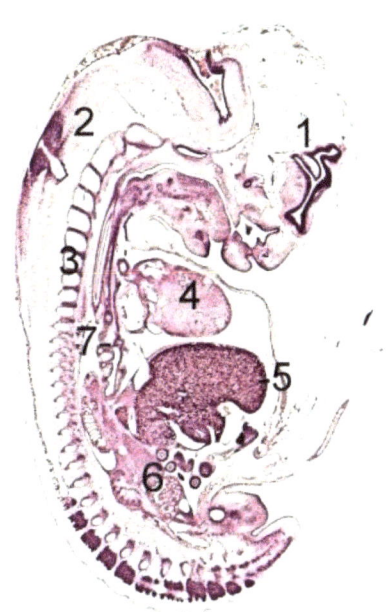

Sheep embryo 26 mm CRL, longitudinal section, HE: 1 brain, 2 spinal cord, 3 vertebral column, 4 heart, 5 liver, 6 mesonephros, 7 lung.

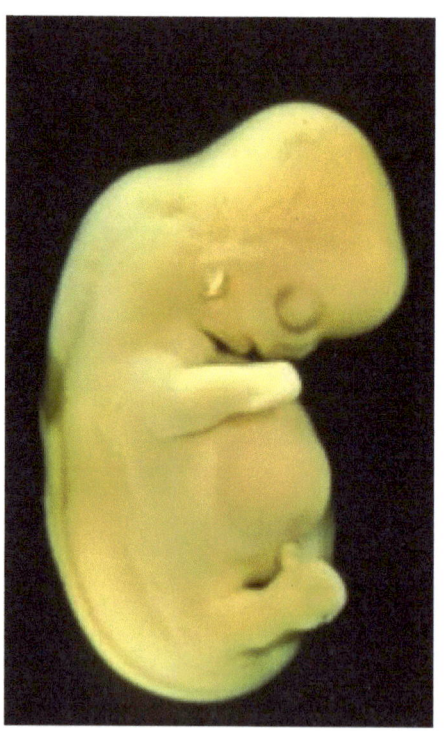

Sheep embryo 28 mm CRL

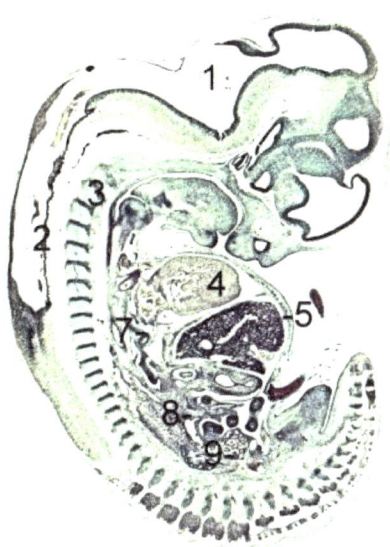

Sheep embryo 28 mm CRL, longitudinal section, HE: 1 rhombencephalon, 2 spinal cord, 3 vertebral column, 4 heart, 5 liver, 7 lung, 8 intestines, 9 mesonephros.

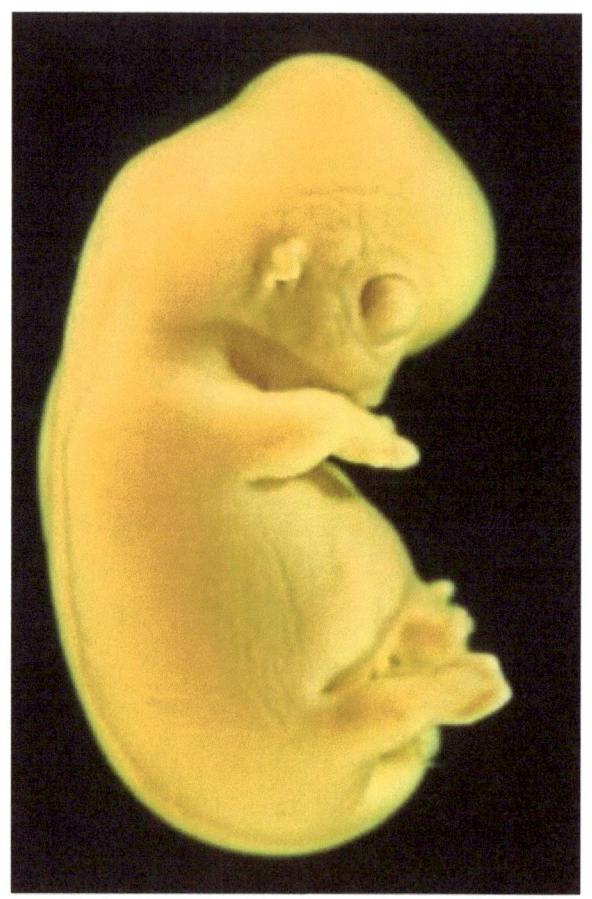

Sheep embryo 31 mm CRL

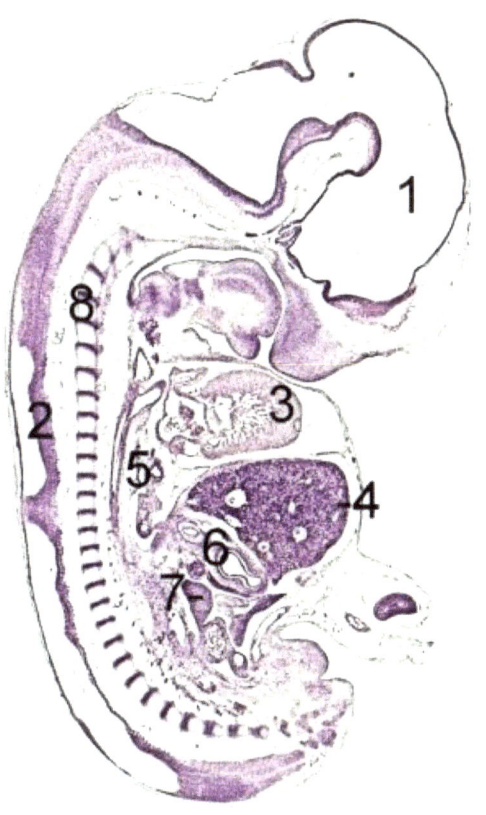

Sheep embryo 31 mm CRL, longitudinal section, HE: 1 brain, 2 spinal cord, 3 heart, 4 liver, 5 lung, 6 stomach, 7 gonad, 8 vertebral column.

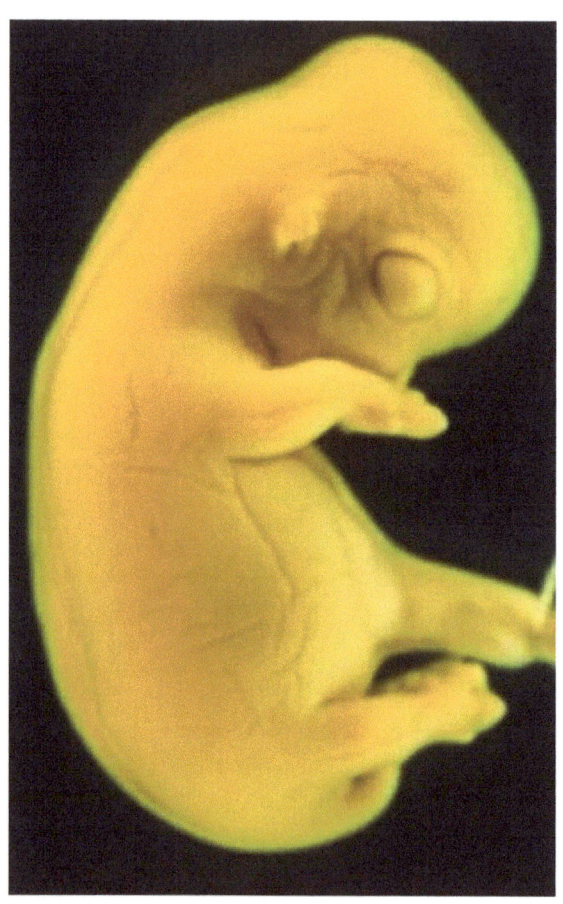

Sheep embryo 34 mm CRL

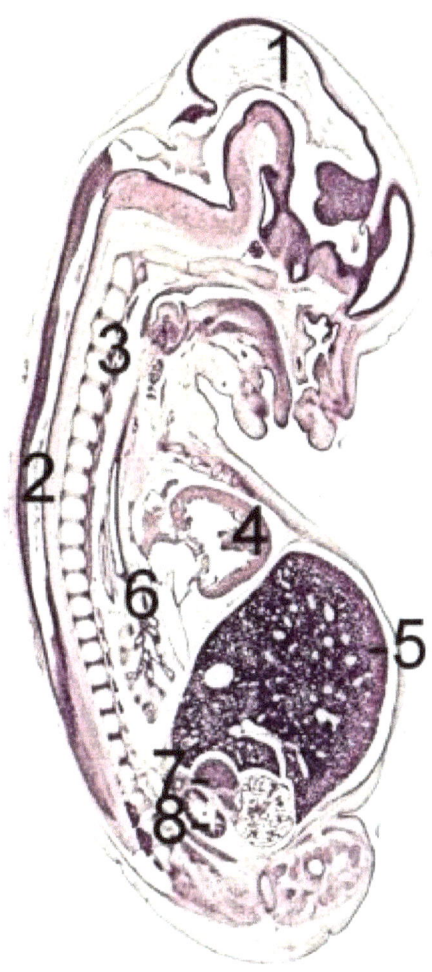

Sheep embryo 36 mm CRL, longitudinal section, HE: 1 brain, 2 spinal cord, 3 vertebral column, 4 heart, 5 liver, 6 lung, 7 gonad, 8 metanephros.

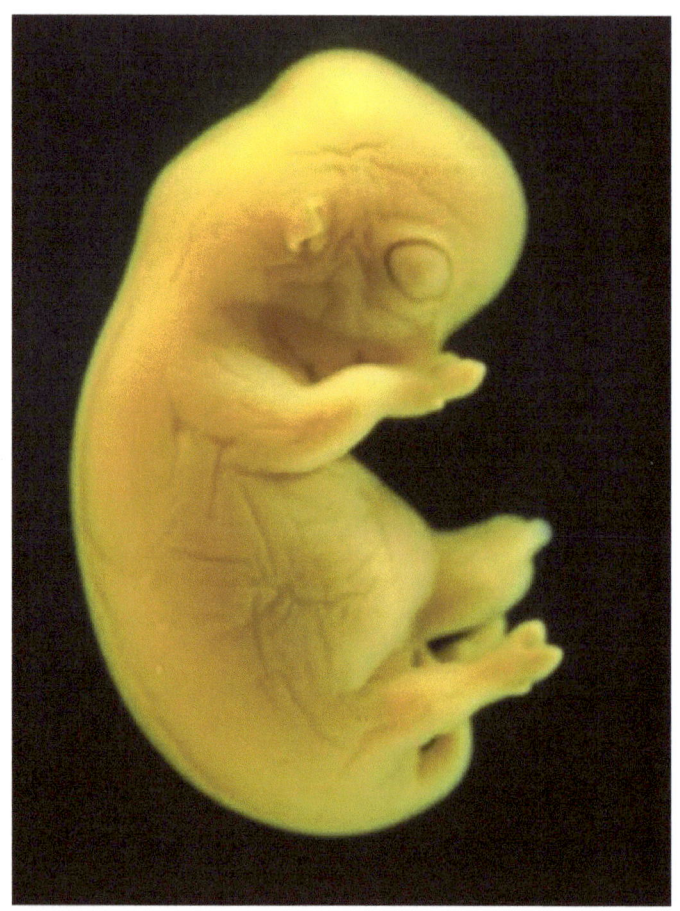

Sheep embryo 38 mm CRL

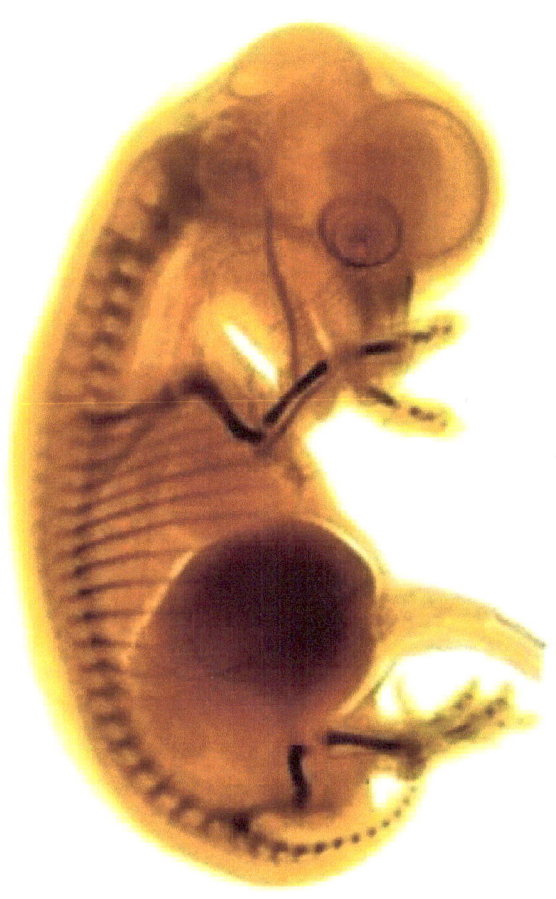

Sheep embryo 41 mm CRL, with cartilage skeleton stained.

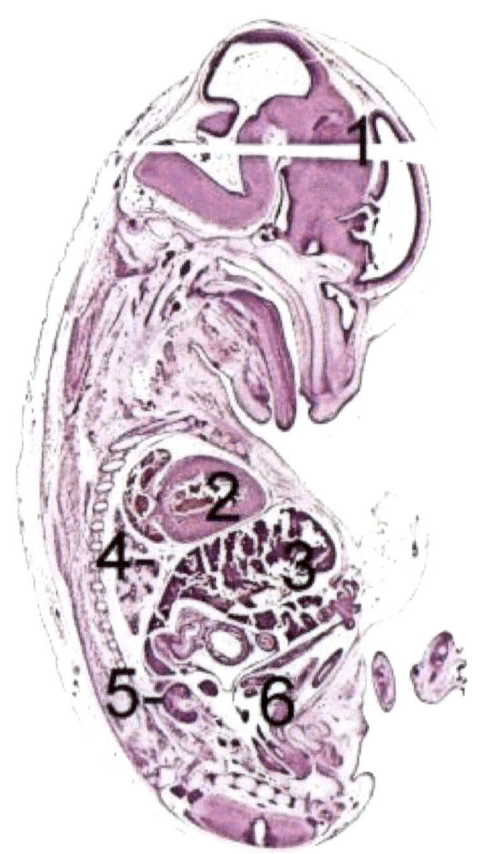

Sheep embryo 43 mm CRL, longitudinal section, HE: 1 brain, 2 heart, 3 liver, 4 lung, 5 kidney, 6 intestines.

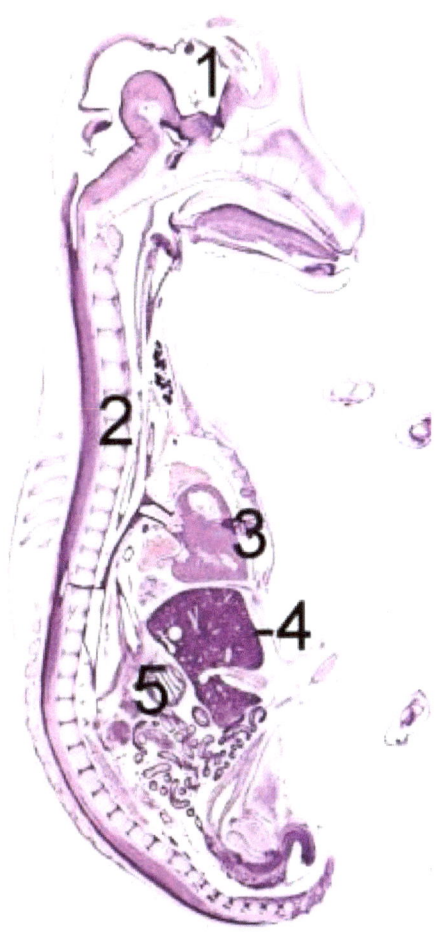

Sheep fetus 60 mm CRL, longitudinal section, HE: 1 brain, 2 spinal cord and vertebrae, 3 heart, 4 liver, 5 stomach.

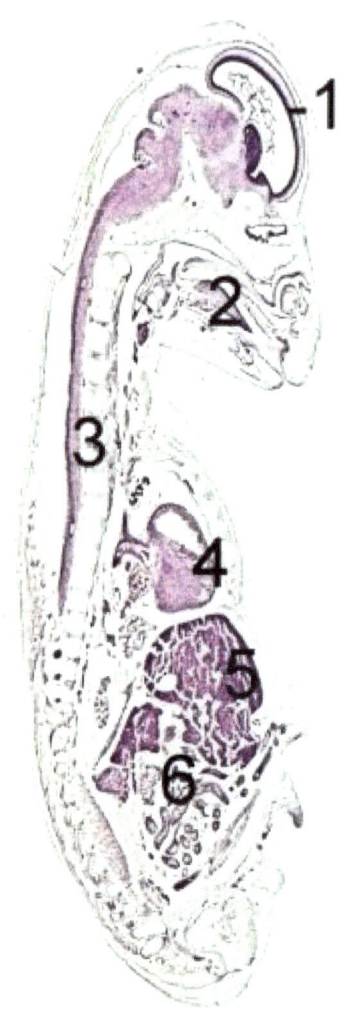

Sheep fetus 65 mm CRL, longitudinal section, GRA: 1 brain, 2 oral cavity, 3 spinal cord and vertebrae, 4 heart, 5 liver, 6 intestines.

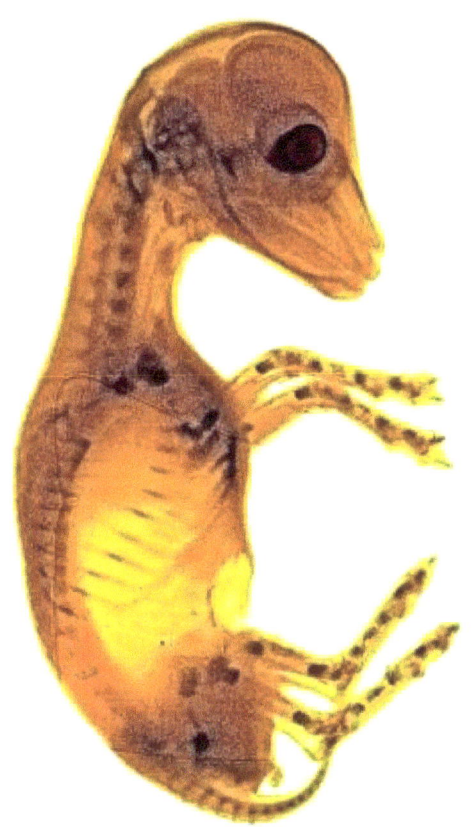

Sheep fetus 88 mm CRL, with stained ossification centers.

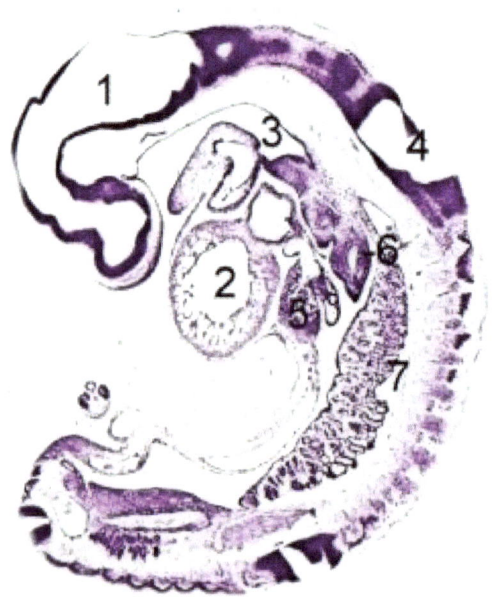

Pig embryo 20 mm CRL, longitudinal section, HE: 1 deuterencephalon, 2 heart, 3 primitive pharynx, 4 neural tube, 5 liver, 6 stomach, 7 mesonephros.

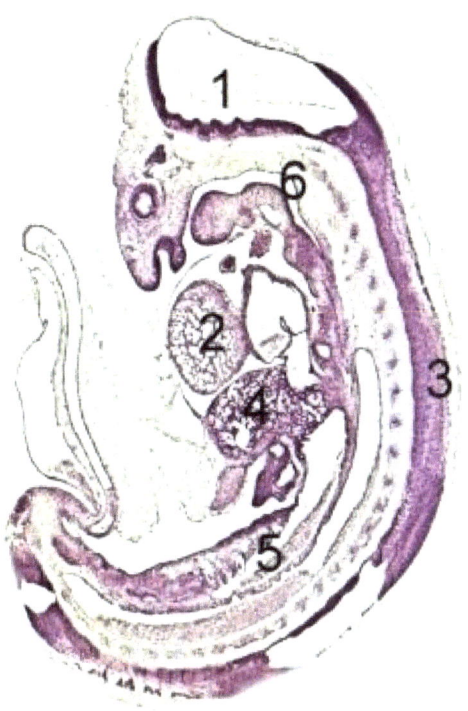

Pig embryo 22 mm CRL, longitudinal section, HE: 1 rhombencephalon, 2 heart, 3 neural tube, 4 liver, 5 mesonephros, 6 pharynx.

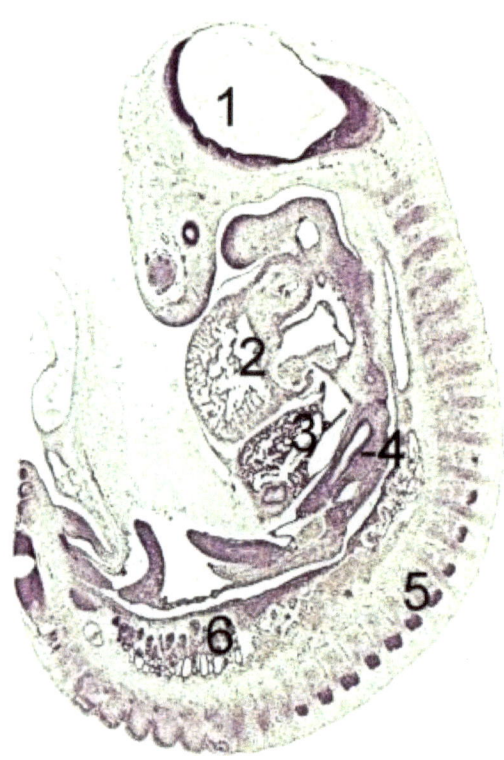

Pig embryo 24 mm CRL, longitudinal section, HE: 1 rhombencephalon, 2 heart, 3 liver, 4 stomach, 5 spinal ganglia, 6 mesonephros.

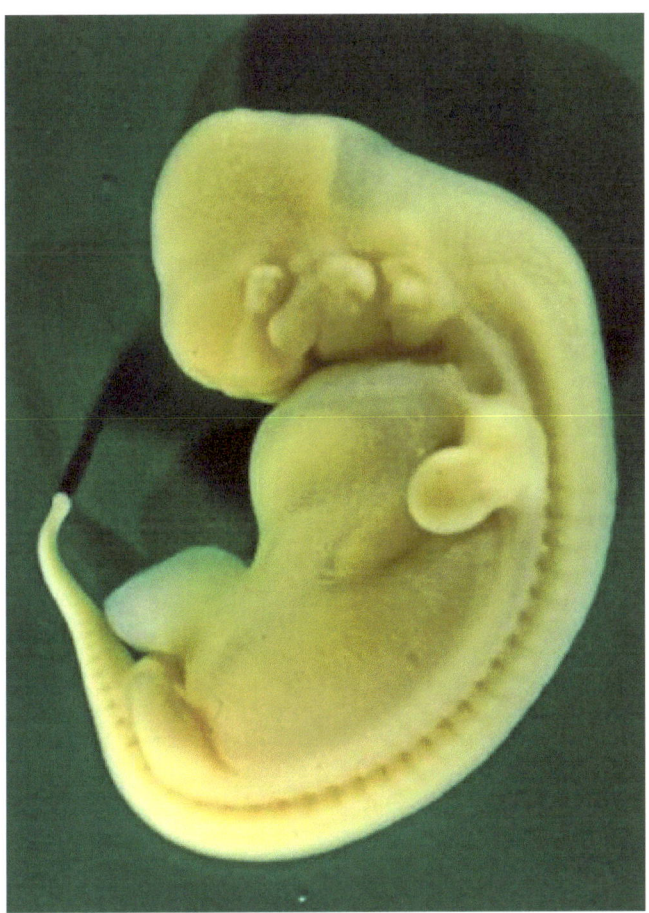

Pig embryo 26 mm CRL

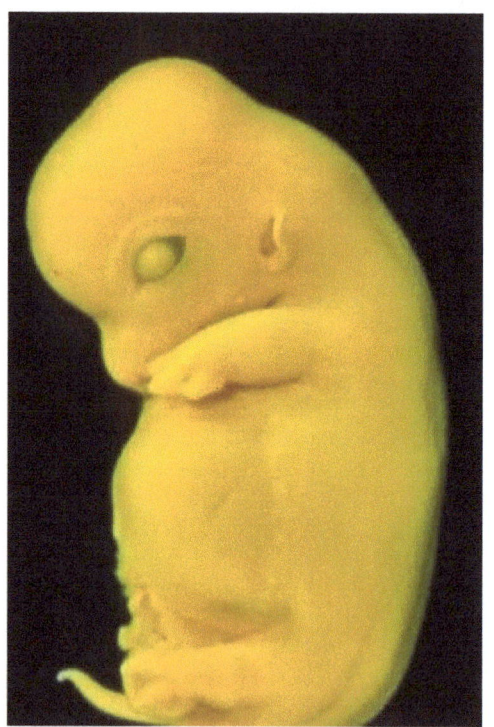
Pig embryo 29 mm CRL

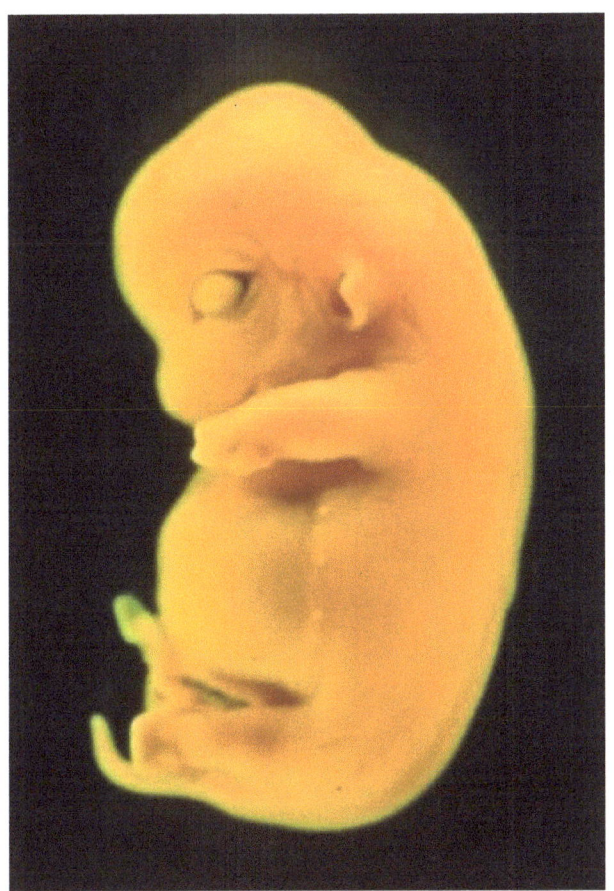

Pig embryo 31 mm CRL

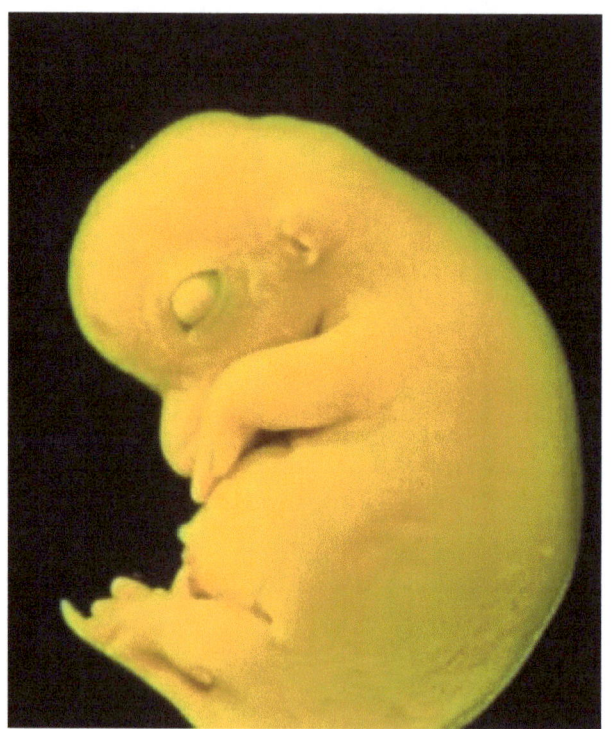

Pig embryo 33 mm CRL

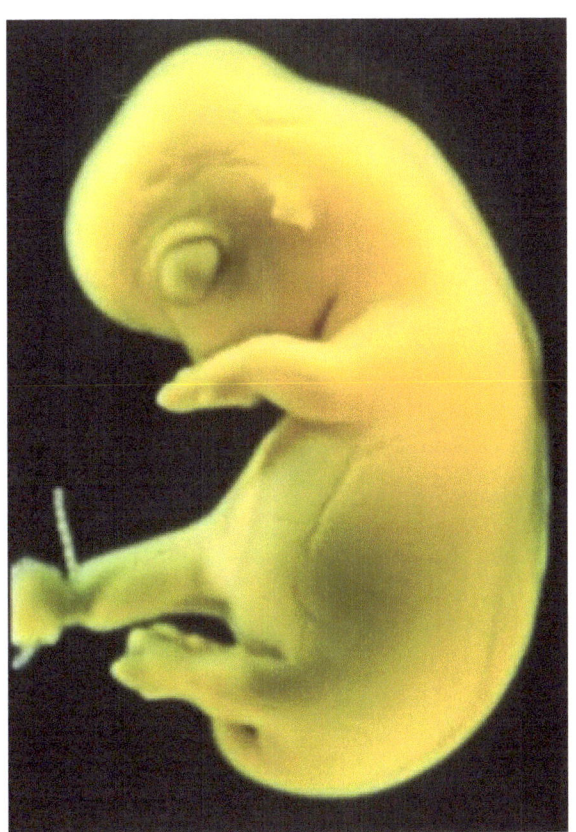

Pig embryo 41 mm CRL

4 SKIN AND DERIVATIVES

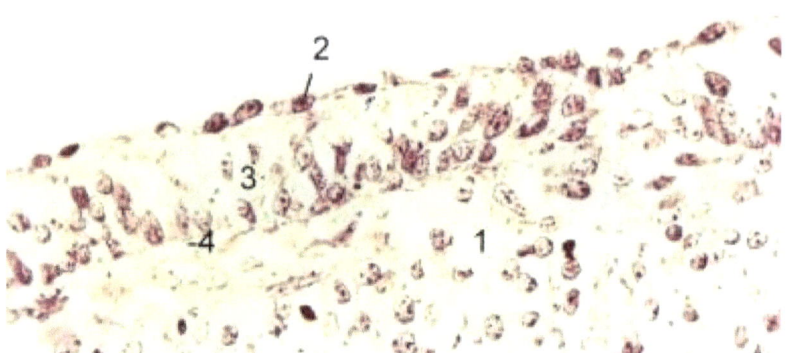

Skin development, abdominal skin, cat embryo, 30 days, cross section, HE, 240x: 1 corium, 2 periderm, 3 epithelial layers, 4 primitive basal membrane.

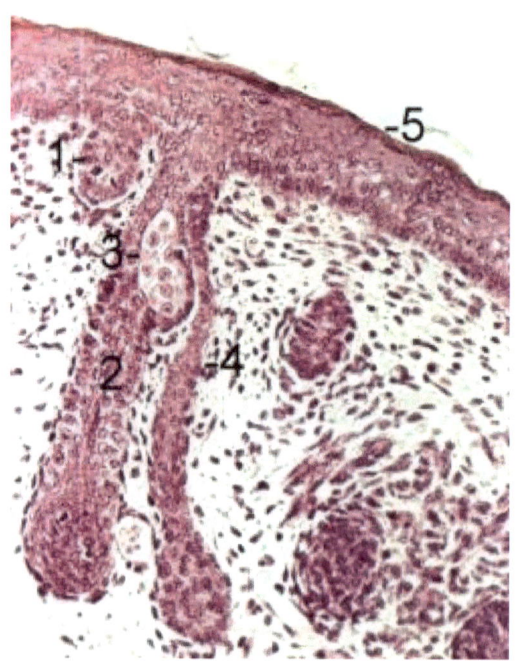

Hair- and gland development, skin of the backside, cat embryo, 53 days, cross section, HE, 95x: 1 hair primordium, 2 club hair, 3 sebaceous gland primordium, 4 sweat gland primordium, 5 periderm.

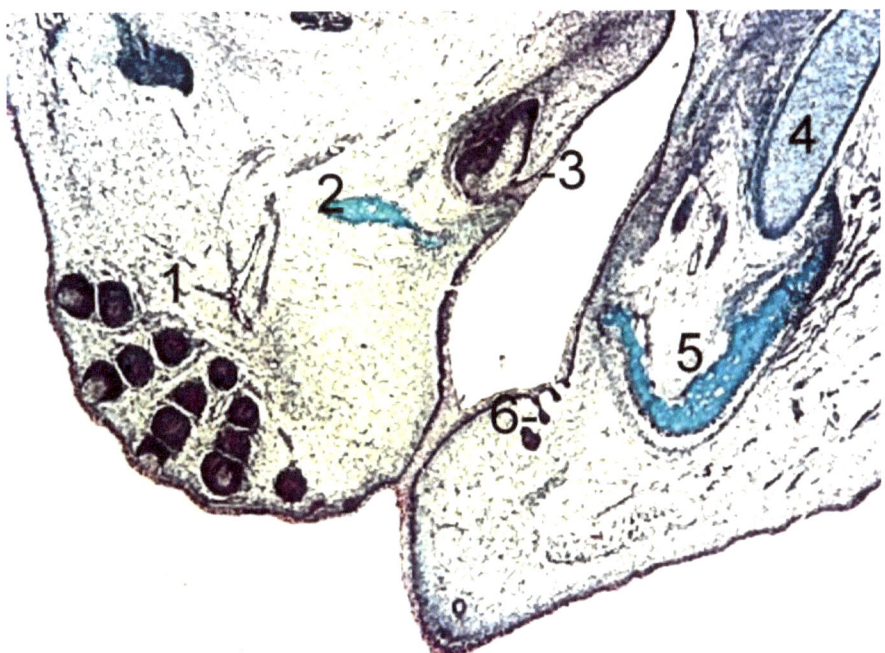

Sinus hairs, Lip cat, 32 days, longitudinal section, GRA, 25x: 1 hair primordia, 2 maxilla, 3 tooth formation in the primitive oral cavity, 4 Meckel's-cartilage, 5 mandibula, 6 salivary glands.

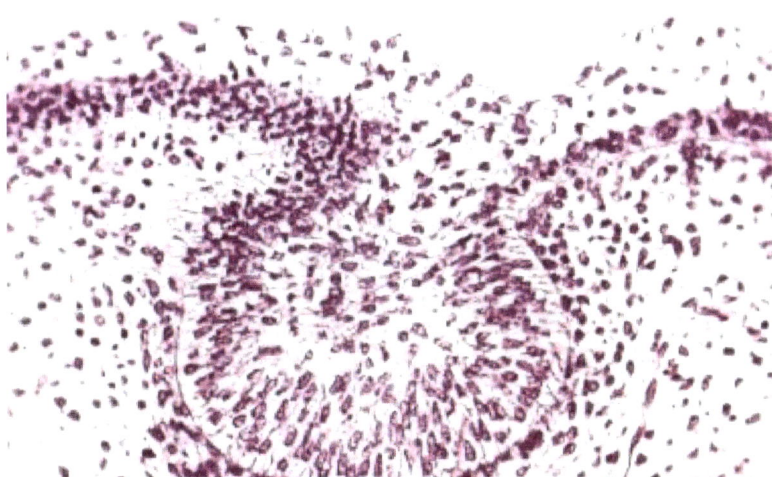

Mammary bud, abdominal skin, sheep embryo, 3 cm CRL, HE, 240x.

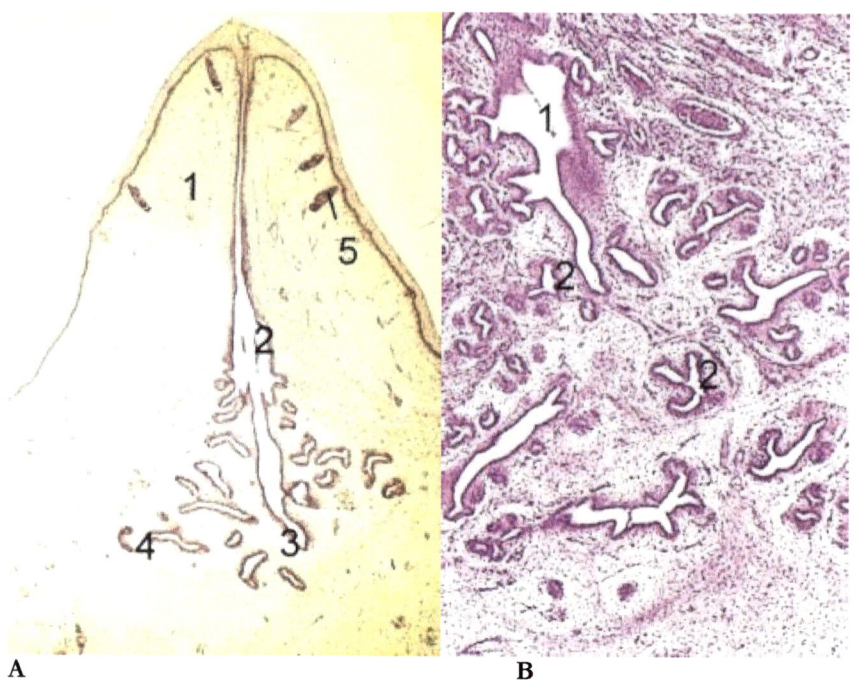

A **B**
Mammary gland development, A teat primordium, sheep embryo, 20 cm CRL, HE, 15x: 1 proliferation papilla, 2 Ductus papillaris and cisterna, 3 primitive lactiferous ducts, 4 solid epithelial sprouts, 5 hairs; **B** udder, sheep embryo, 30 cm CRL, HE, 15x: 1 cistern, 2 primitive lactiferous ducts.

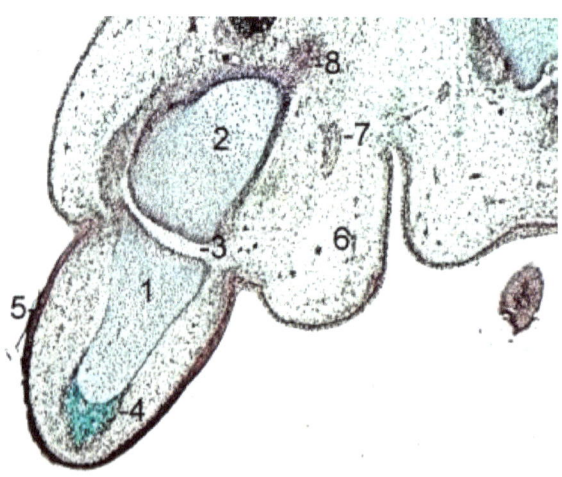

Claw development, cat embryo, 34 Tage, GRA, 15x: 1/2 cartilage of the phalanges, 3 primordium of the phalageal joint, 4 intramembranous ossification of the claw, 5 paries of the claw, 6 pad of the claw, 7 nerve, 8 extensory tendon.

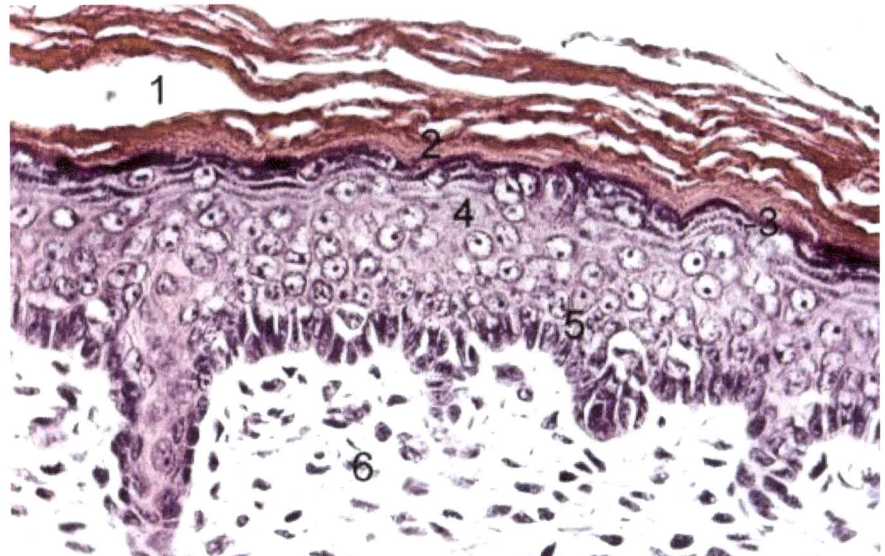

Keratinization, digital pad, cat embryo, 53 days, HE, 375x: 1 Stratum corneum, 2 Stratum lucidum, 3 Stratum granulosum, 4 Stratum spinosum, 5 Stratum germinativum, 6 papillary body.

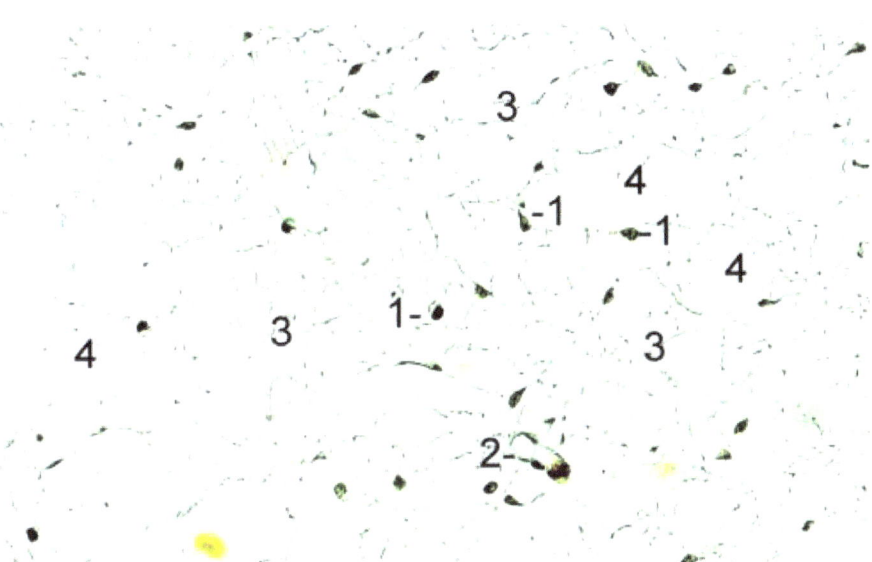

Mesenchyme, cat embryo, GRA, 240x: 1 mesenchyme cells, 2 capillaries, embryonal fibers, 4 ground substance.

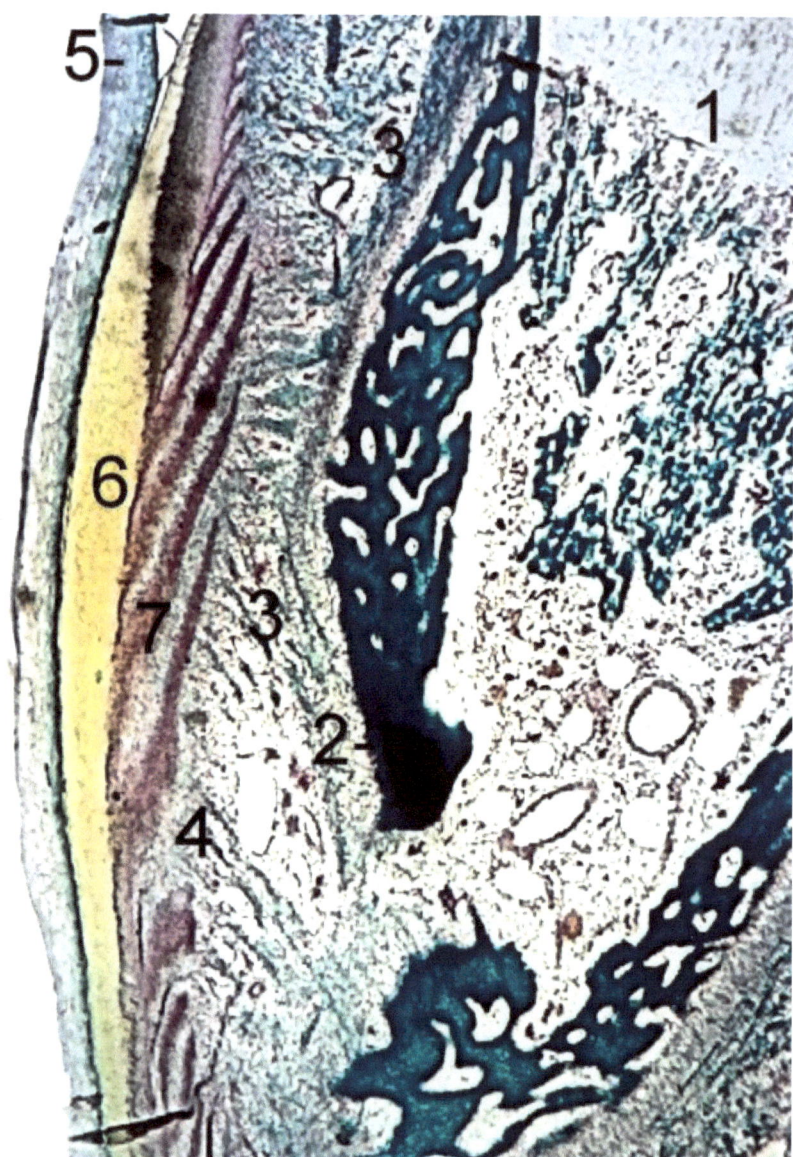

Claw, sheep, last trimester, longitudinal, GRA, 25x: 1 cartilage of the distal phalanx and its endochondral ossification, 2 intramembranous ossification of the distal phalangeal tip, 3 dermis, 4 dermal papillae, 5 limbic keratin, 6 coronal keratin, 7 epidermal papillae.

5 LOCOMOTIV APPARATUS

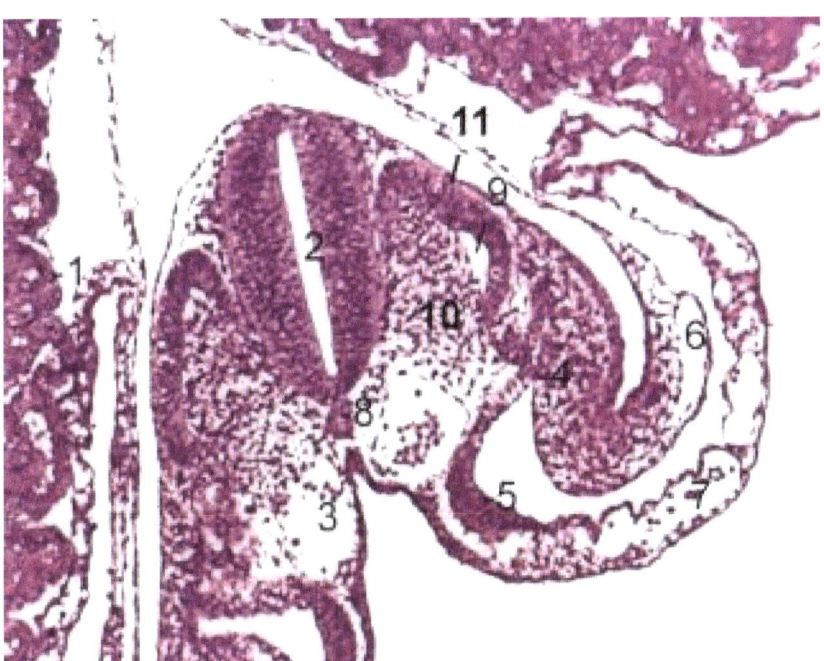

Somite differentiation, cat embryo, 19 days, cross section, HE, 95x: 1 placenta, 2 neural tube, 3 aorta, 4 somite stalk, 5 mesothel, 6 somatopleura, 7 visceropleura, 8 notochord, 9 somitocoeloma, 10 sclerotom, 11 dermatomyotom.

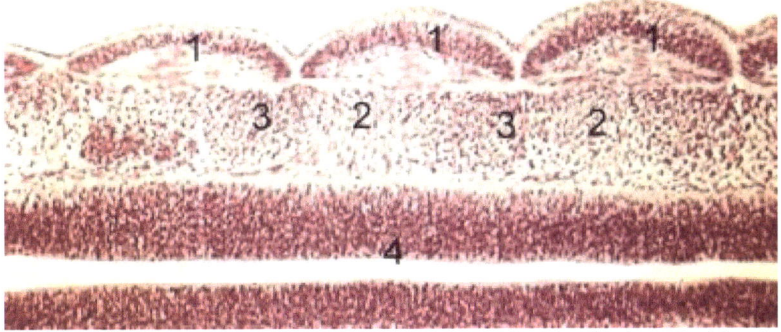

Vertebral primordium, cat embryo, 17 days, longitudinal, HE, 95x: 1 dermatomyotom, cranial part (2) and caudal part (3) of the sclerotomes connected to the primordia of the vertebrae, 4 neural tube.

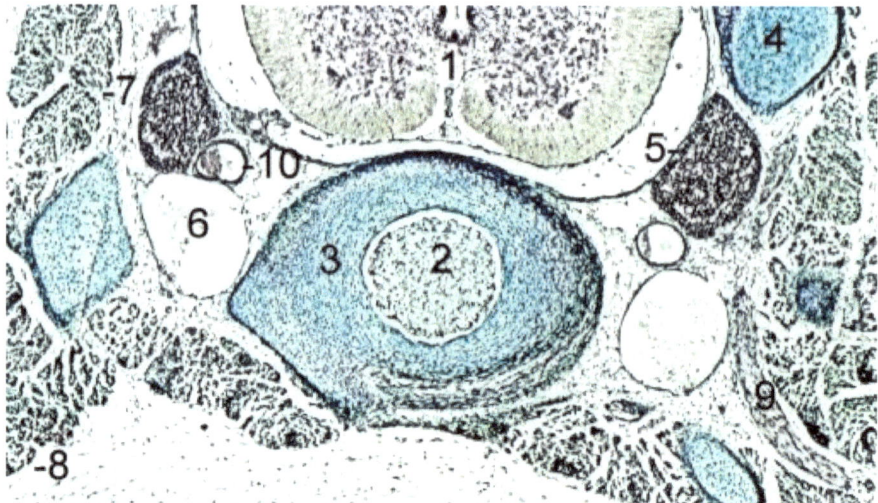

Cartilage skeleton, cat embryo, 34 days, cross section, GRA, 25x: 1 primordium of the spinal cord, 2 remnants of the notochord, 3 cartilaginous body, 5 spinal ganglion, 6 spinal veins, 7 epaxial myoblasts, 8 hypaxial myoblasts, 9 spinal nerve, 10 vertebral artery.

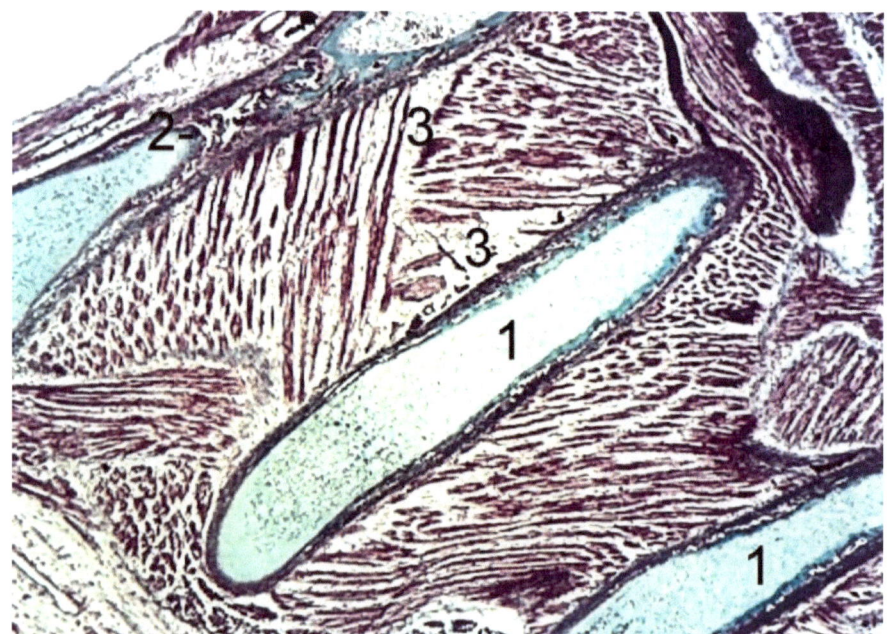

Rip development, cat embryo, 26 Tage, längs, GRA, 25x: 1 cartilagenous rips, 2 ossification zone, 3 primordium of the intercostal muscles.

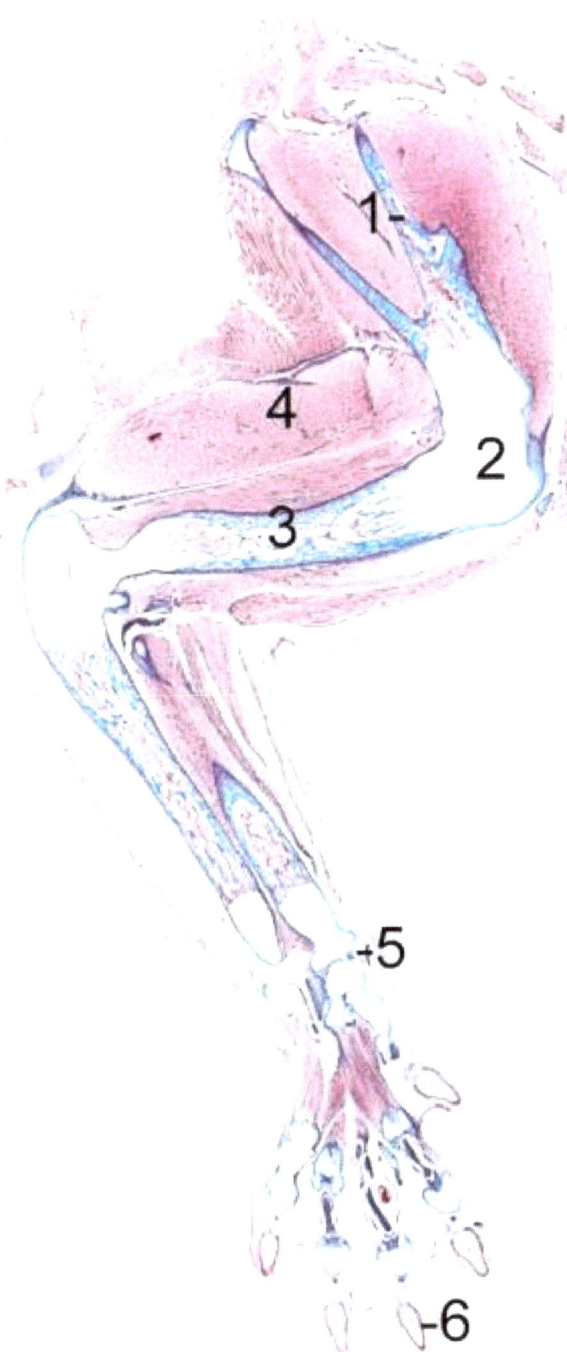

Ossification, pectoral limb, cat embryo, 44 days, longitudinal section, GRA, 12x: 1 intramembranous ossification of the spine of the scapula, 2 epiphyseal cartilage, 3 endochondral ossification of the diaphyse, 4 muscle primodia, 5 joint primordia, 6 keratinization of the claw epidermis.

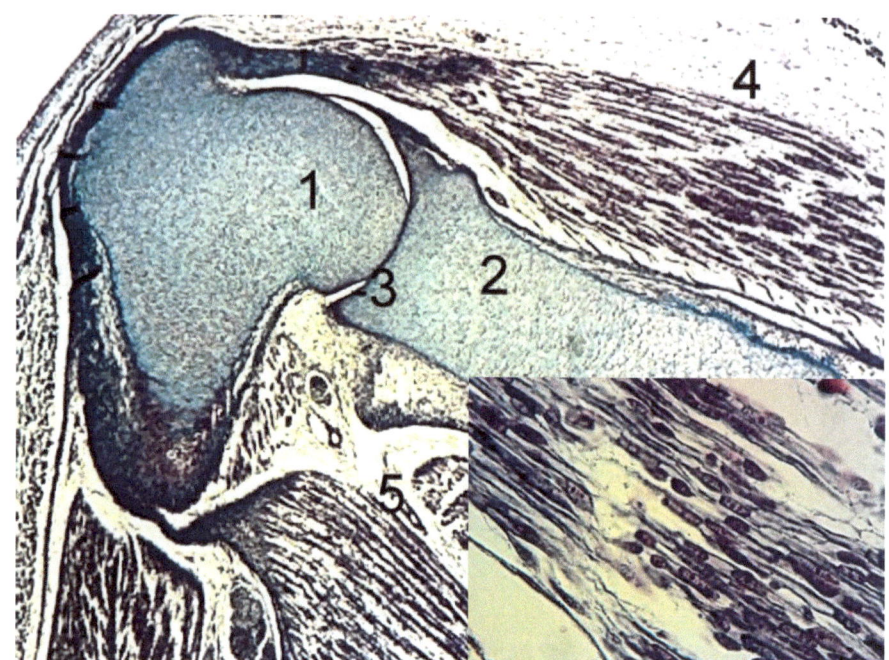

Shoulder joint, cat embryo 32 days, longitudinal, GRA 25x: 1 humeral cartilage, 2 cartilageous scapula, 3 joint primordium, 4 myoblasts of the supraspinatus muscle, 5 myoblasts of the infraspinatus muscle; magnification: fusion of the myoblasts.

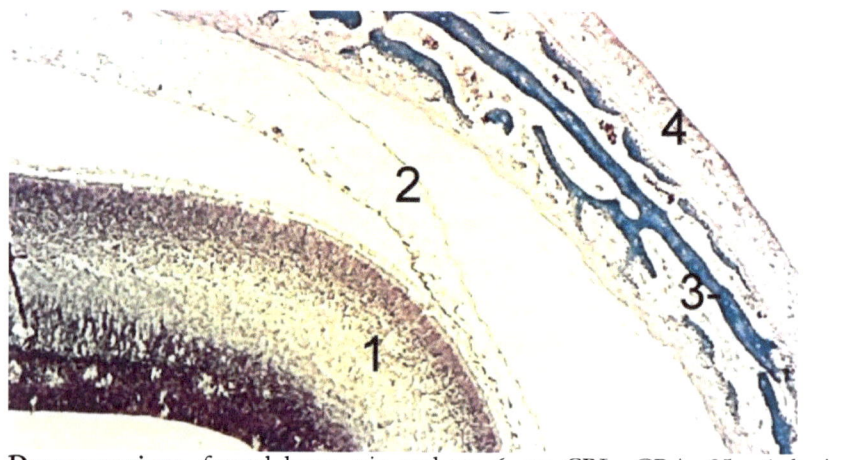

Desmocranium, frontal bone, pig embryo 6 cm CRL, GRA, 25x: 1 brain, 2 primitive meninx, 3 bone, 4 scalp.

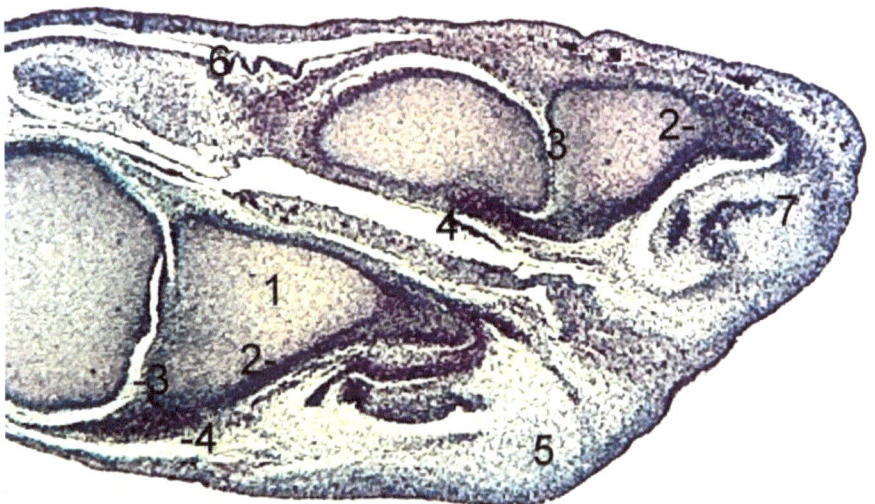

Paw development, cat embryo 7 cm CRL, GRA, 15x: 1 cartilagenous proximal phalanx, 2 intramembranous ossification of the distal phalanx, 3 phalangeal joints, 4 ligaments, 5 digital pad, 6 extensory tendon, 7 developing claw.

6 CIRCULATORY SYSTEM

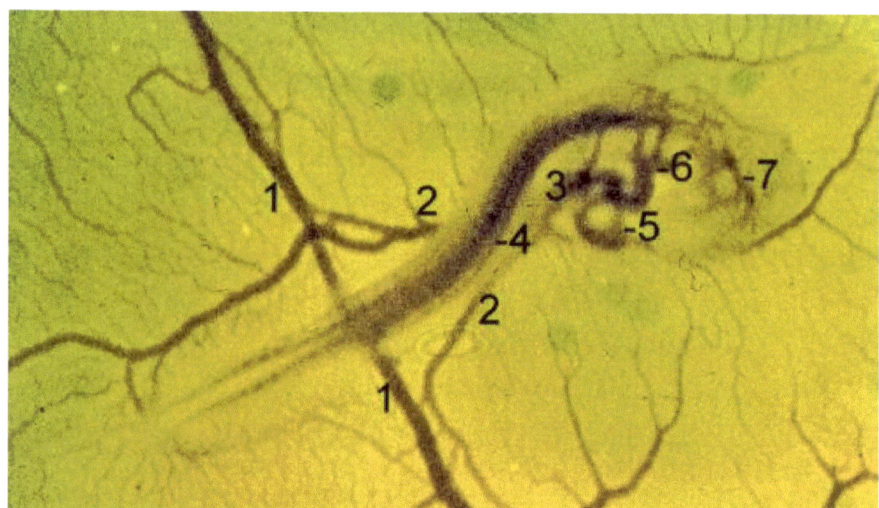

Vitelline circulation, duck embryo, 3 days, unstained, 15x: 1 Aa. omphalomesentericae (vitellinae), 2 Vv. omphalomesentericae, 3 Ductus cuveri and sinus cordis, 4 dorsal aortae, 5 ventricular loop, 6 bulb and arterial trunk, 7 cranial cardinal veins.

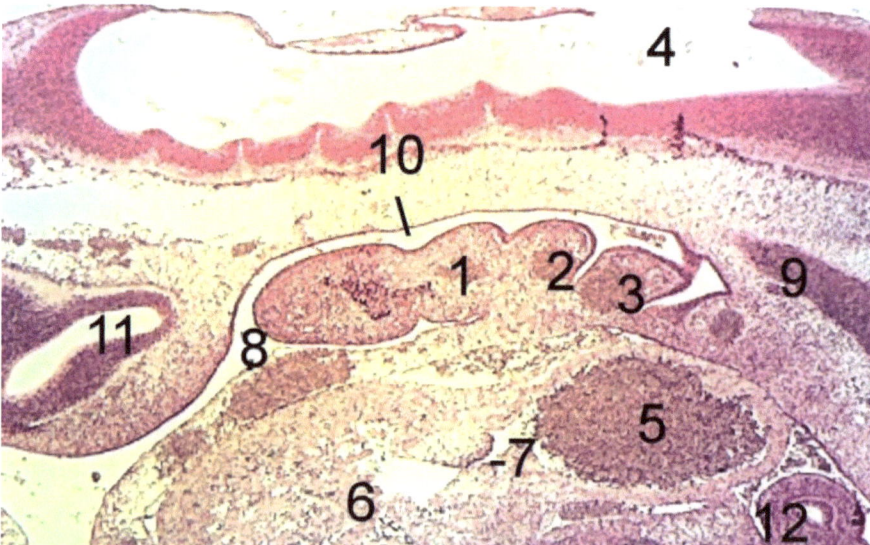

Pharygeal arteries, cattle embryo, 1 cm CRL, longitudinal, HE, 25x: 1 1st pharyngeal artery, 2 second, 3 third, 4 rhombencephalon, 5 bulb of the heart, 6 ventricle, 7 endocardial cushion, 8 primitive stomodaeum, 9 dorsal aortae, 10 primitiv pharynx, 11 forebrain vesicle, 12 gastric primordium.

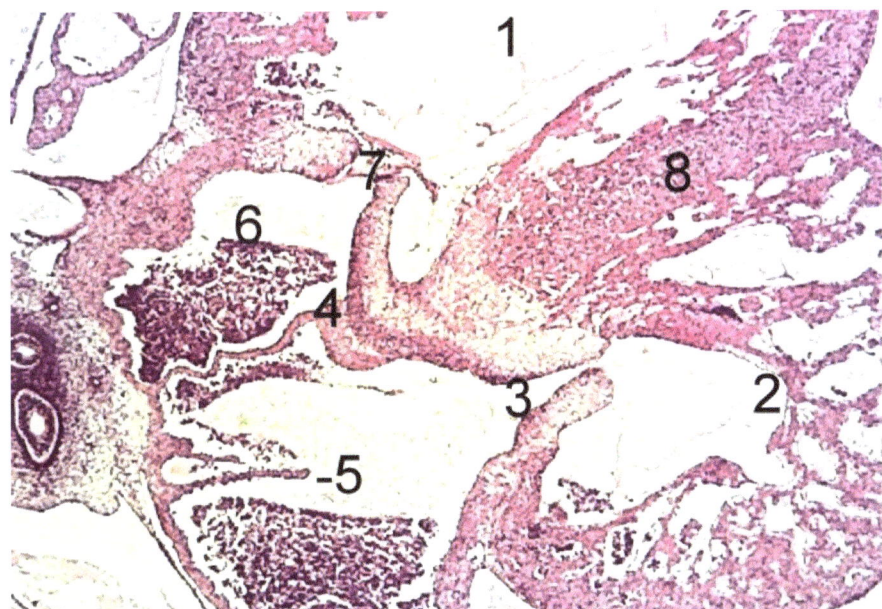

Septation of the heart, sheep embryo, 2cm CRL, cross, HE, 25x: 1 left-, 2 right ventricle, 3 atrioventricular ostium, 4 primary septum, 5 Septum secundum, 6 left atrium, 7 valve, 8 interventricular septum.

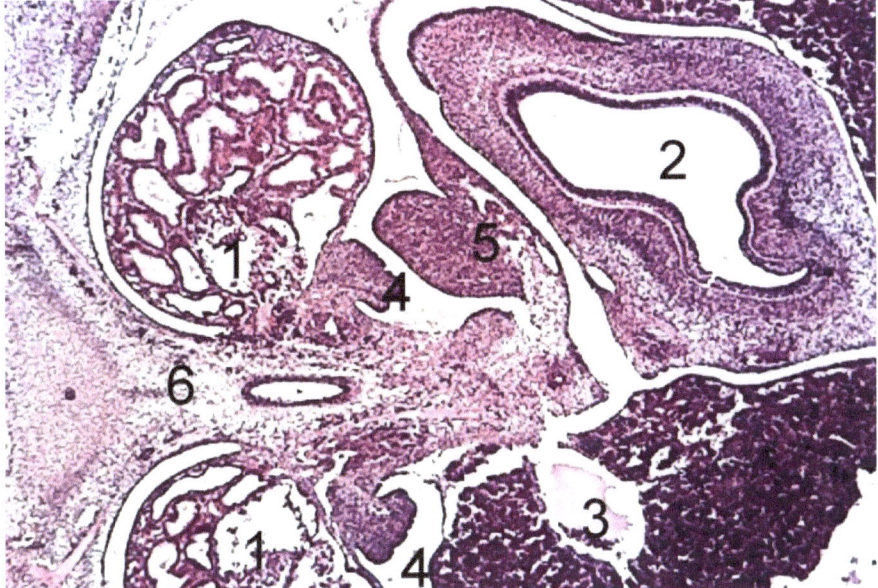

Spleen primordium, sheep embryo, 2cm CRL, quer, HE, 25x: 1 mesonephros, 2 stomach, 3 liver, 4 suprarenal, 5 spleen inside the dorsal mesogastrium, 6 mesentry.

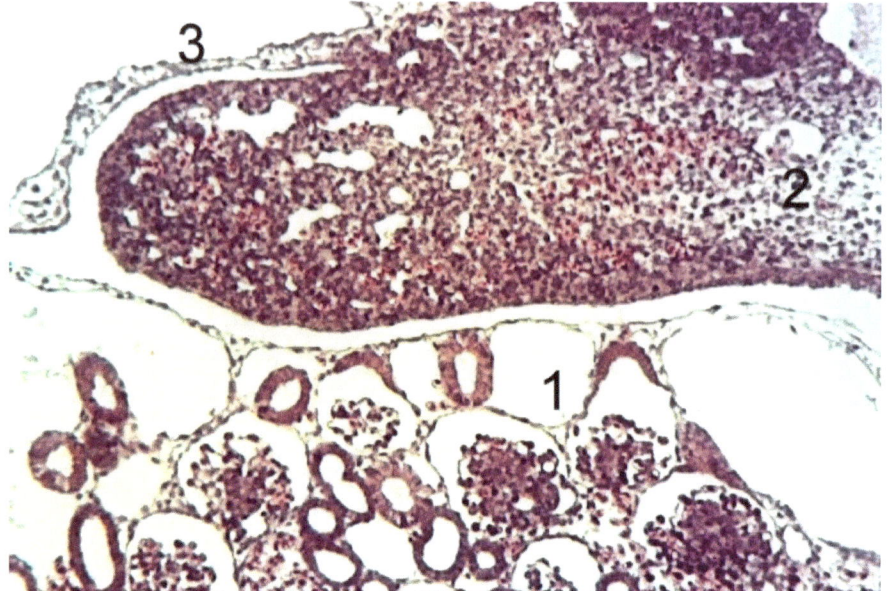

Spleen, dog embryo, 6 days, cross, GRA, 25x: 1 mesonephros, 2 spleen with capillaries, 3 dorsal mesogastrium.

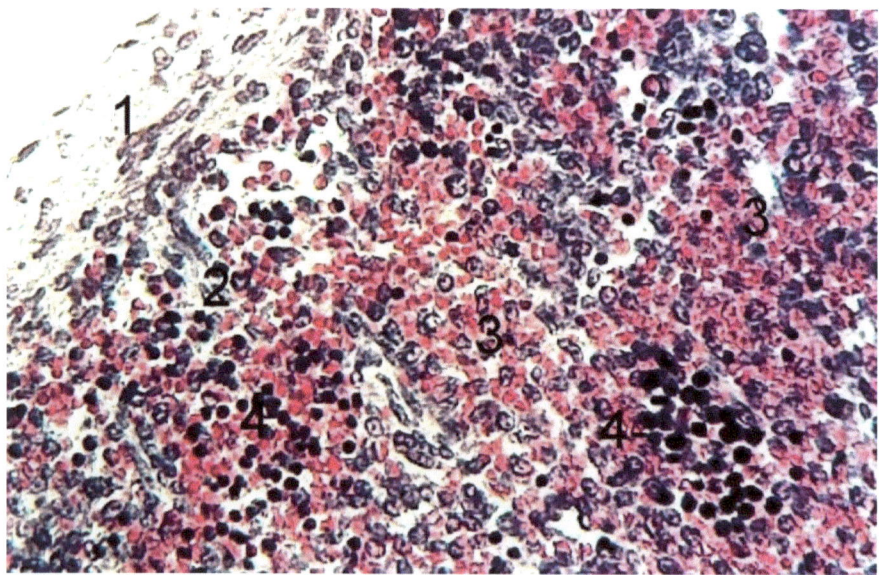

Primordium of the pulp, spleen, sheep embryo 10cm CRL, GRA, 240x: 1 capsule, 2 trabecle, 3 red pulp primordium, 4 white pulp primordium with haematopoiesis.

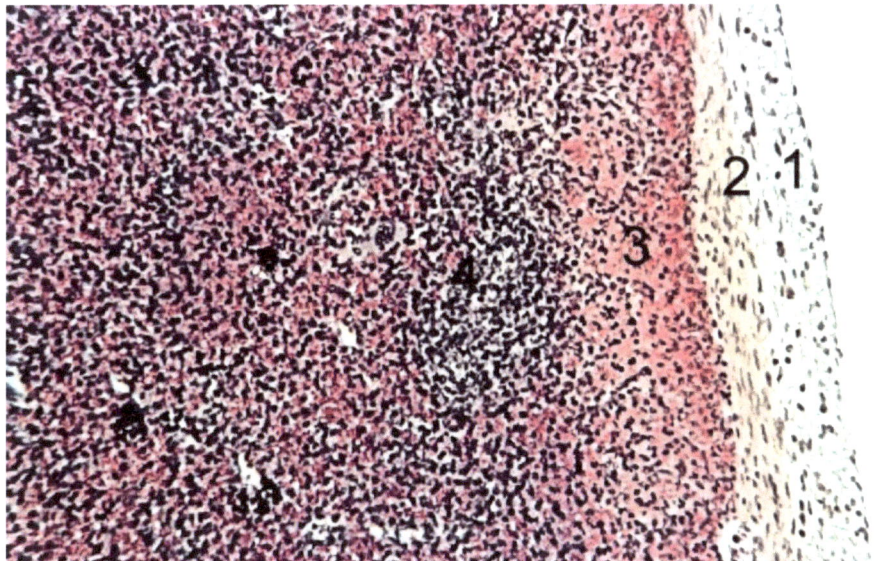

Differentiation of the spleen, sheep embryo, 44 CRL, GRA, 95x: 1 fibrous capsule, 2 smooth muscle cells, 3 trabecles, 4 white pulp.

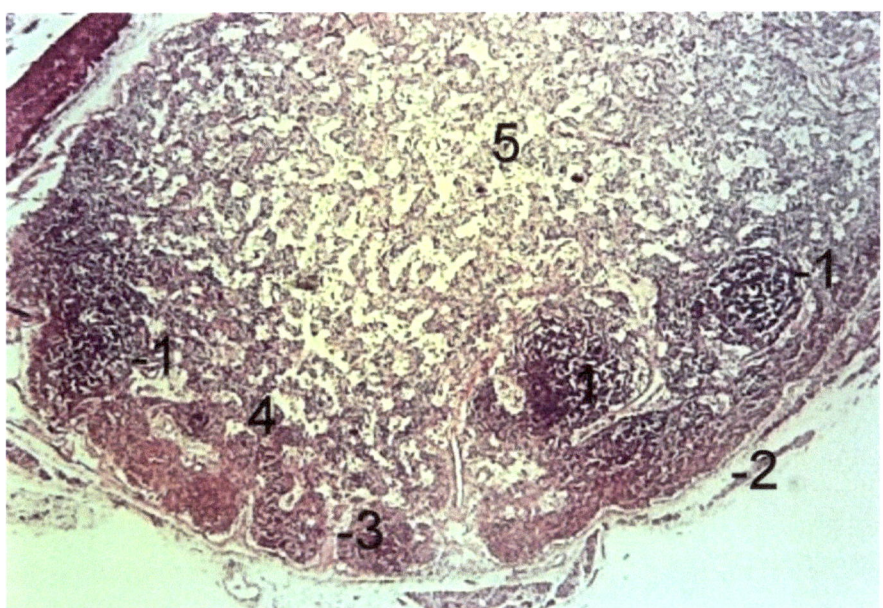

Development of lymphatic nodes, dog embryo, 19 cm CRL, HE, 25x: 1 primary follicles, 2 capsule, 3 trabecle, 4 cortex, 5 medulla.

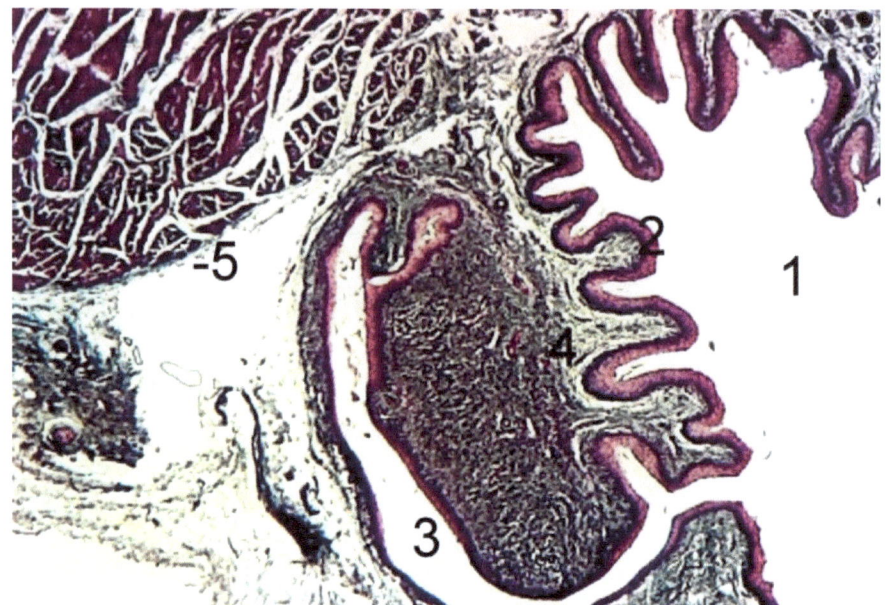

Development of tonsills, pharnygeal tonsil, longitudinal, dog embryo 19cm CRL, GRA, 25x: 1 pharyngeal cavity, 2 mucosa, 3 tonsilar sinus, 4 primordium of the tonsil, 5 pharyngeal muscles.

7 RESPIRATORY APPARATUS

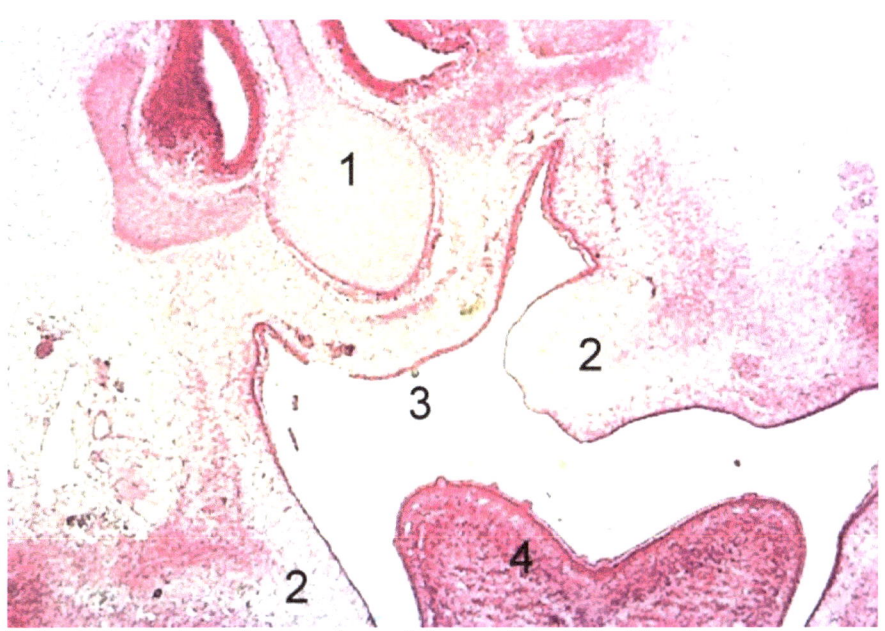

Palatal formation, sheep embryo, 3,5 cm CRL, HE, 25x: 1 nasal septum, 2 secundary palatal processes, 3 nasal- and oral cavity, 4 tongue.

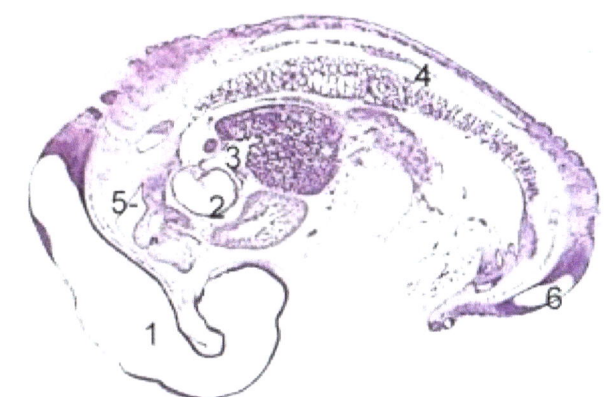

Laryngotracheal groove, pig embryo, 20 mm, longitudinal, HE, 25x: 1 brain vesicle, 2 heart, 3 liver, 4 mesonephros, 5 laryngotracheal groove, 6 neural tube.

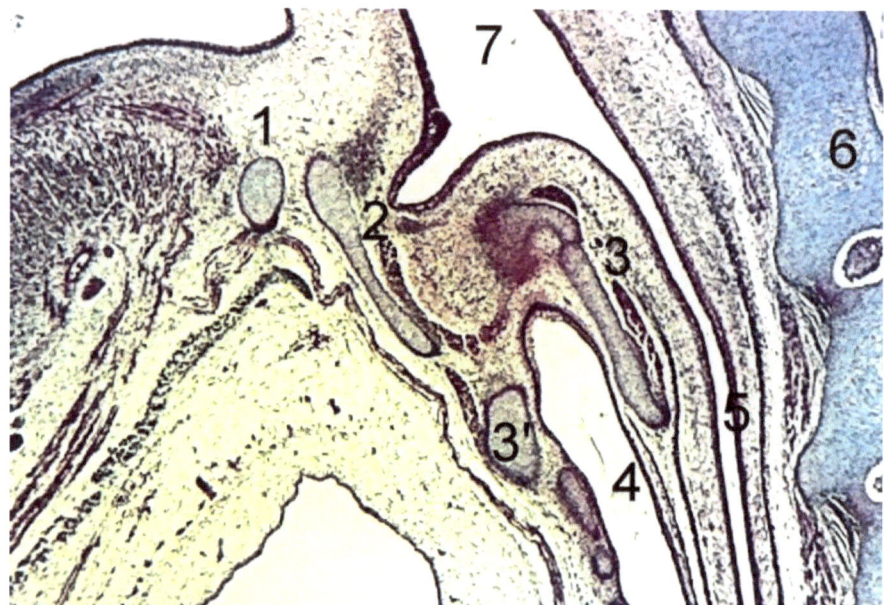

Larynx development, cat embryo, 32 days, GRA, 25x: 1 hyoid, 2 thyreoid cartilage, 3 cricoid plate, 3' cricoid ring, 4 trachea, 5 oesophagus, 6 vertebrae, 7 pharynx.

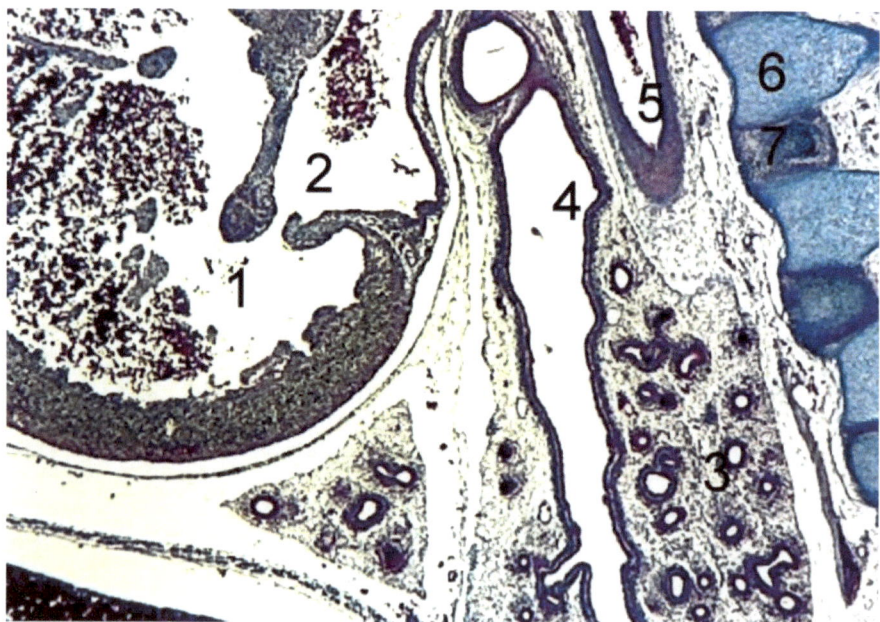

Early lung development, cat embryo, 28 days, GRA, 25x: 1 heart, 2 Bulb, 3 lung during pseudoglandular stage, 4 trachea, 5 aorta, 6 vertebrae, 7 discus.

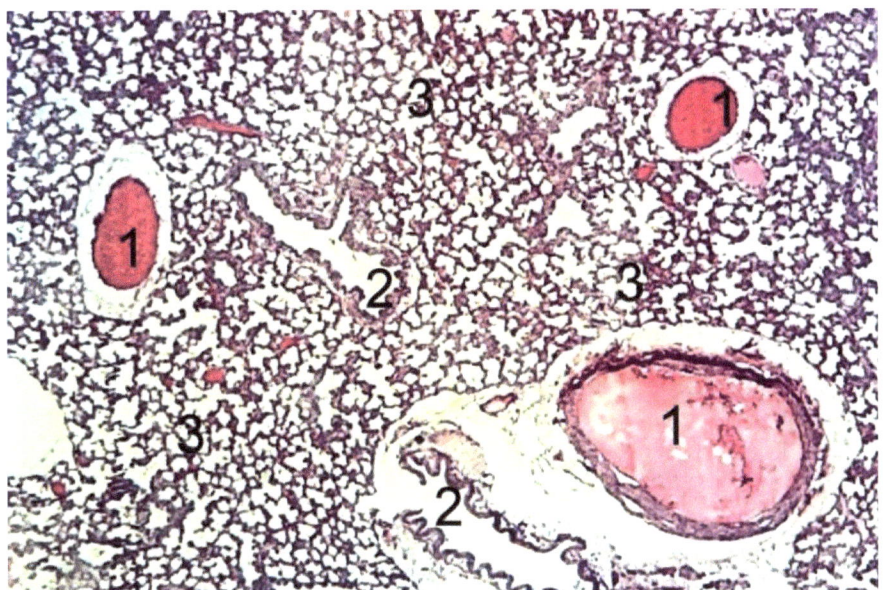

Late lung development, dog embryo, 19 cm CRL, GRA, 25x: 1 lung vessels, 2 bronchial tree, 3 terminal sacs and canaliculi.

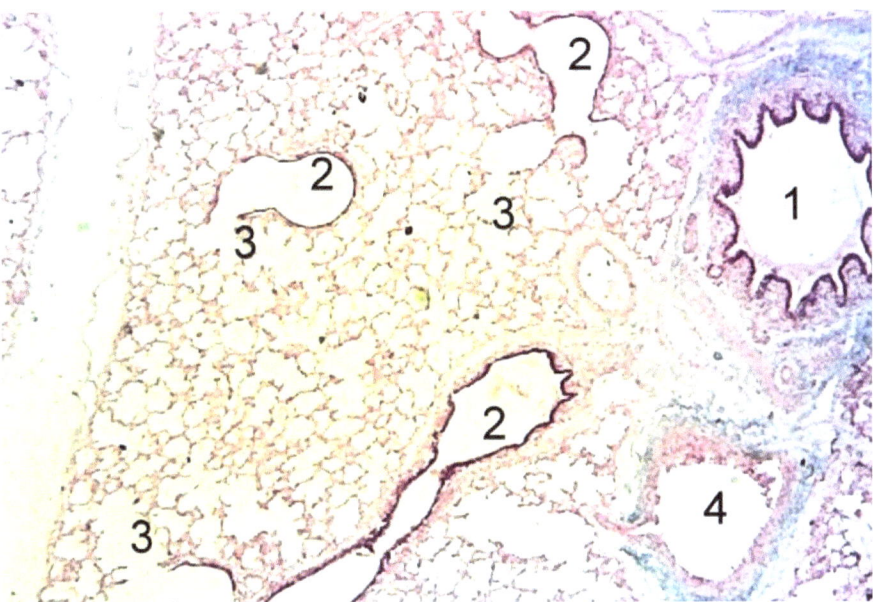

Maturing lung, pig embryo, prenatal, GRA, 25x: 1 bronchus, 2 bronchiolus, 3 first alveols, 4 bronchial vessels.

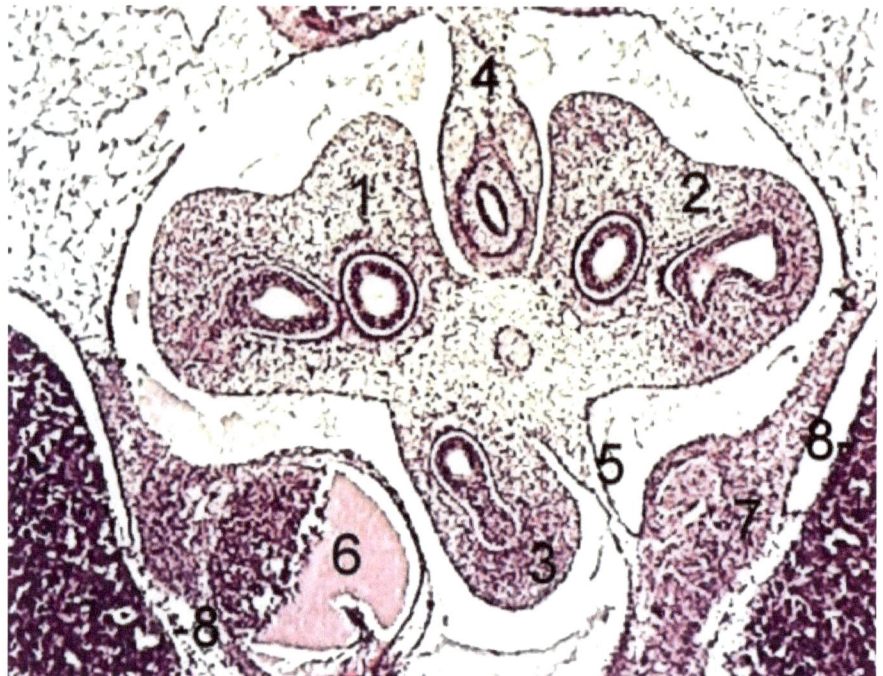

Mediastinal development, sheep embryo 2 cm CRL, HE, 25x: 1 right lung, 2 left lung, 3 accessory lobe, 4 dorsal mesentry of the oesophagus, 5 mediastinum, 6 caudal caval vein, 7 diaphragm, 8 liver.

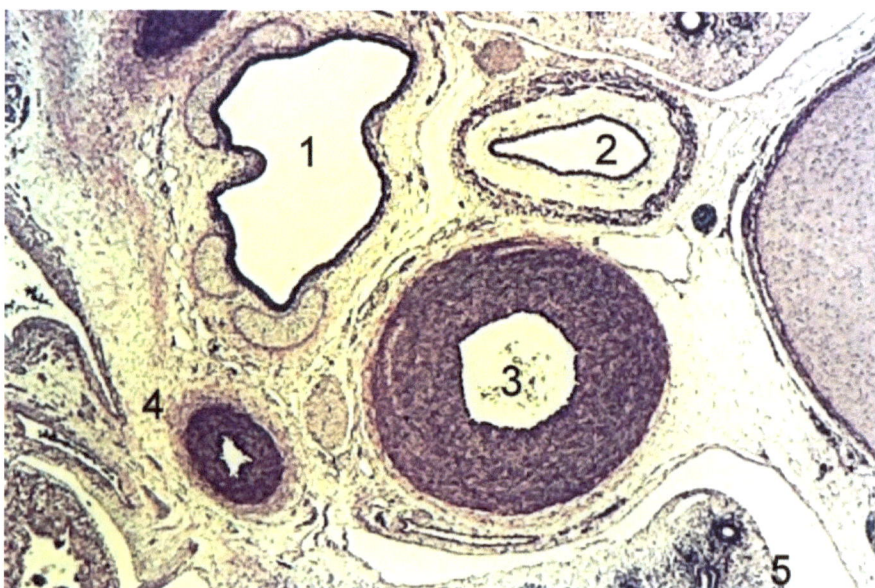

Bifurcatio, pig embryo, 6 cm CRL, GRA, 25x: 1 bifurcation, 2 oesophagus, 3 aorta, 4 pulmonary artery, 5 lung.

8 DISGESTORY APPARATUS

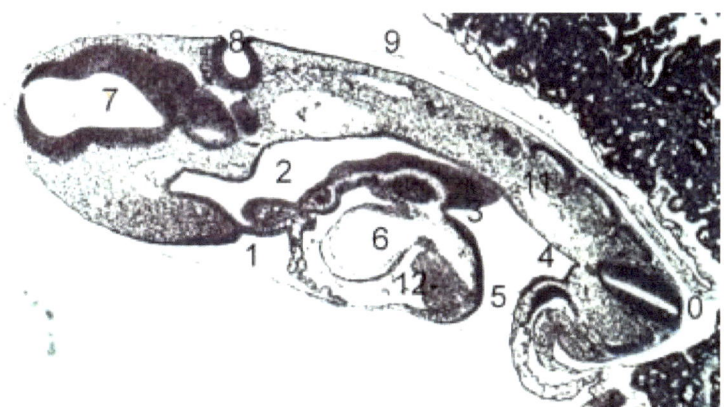

Primitiv gut, cat embryo, 17 days, longitudinal, GRA, 25x: 1 primitive stomodaeum, 2 primitive pharynx, 3 cranial intestinal portal, 4 caudal intestinal portal, 5 Ductus omphaloentericus, 6 heart loop, 7 midbrain vesicle, 8 otic pit, 9 amnion, 10 neural tube, 11 somite, 12 liver plate.

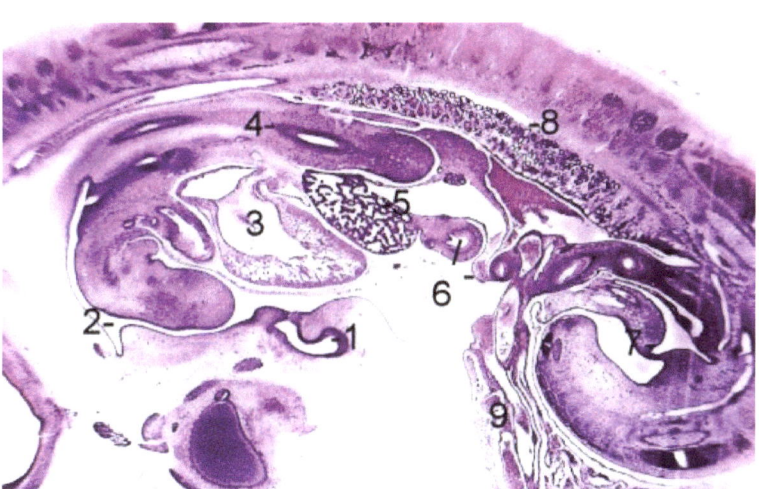

Intestinal tube, duck, 6 days, HE, 15x: 1 nasal pit, 2 primitive pharynx, 3 heart, 4 stomach primordium, 5 liver, 6 primitive intestinal loop, 7 urogenital sinus, 8 mesonephros, 9 yolk sac stalk.

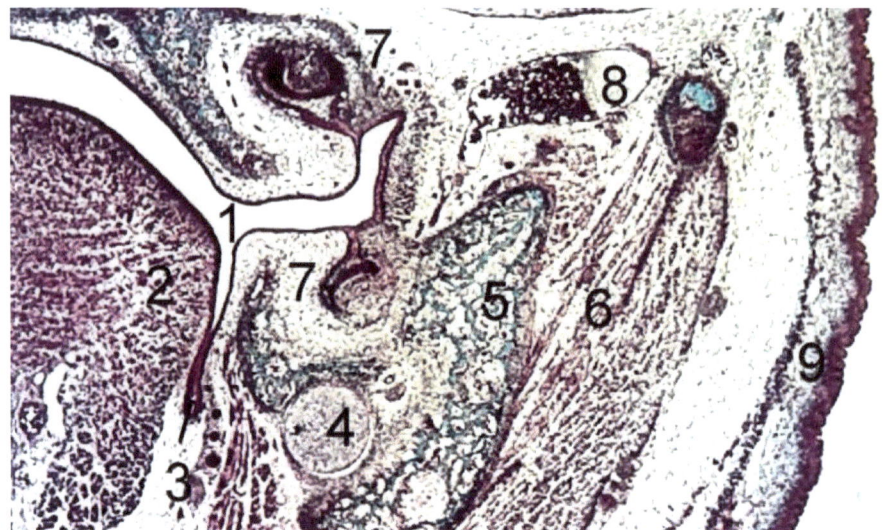

Tooth germs, rat embryo, GRA, 25x: 1 primitive oral cavity, 2 tongue, 3 salivary glands, 4 Meckel's cartilage, 5 mandibular bone, 6 masseter-blastem, 7 tooth germ, 8 maxillary vein, 9 skin.

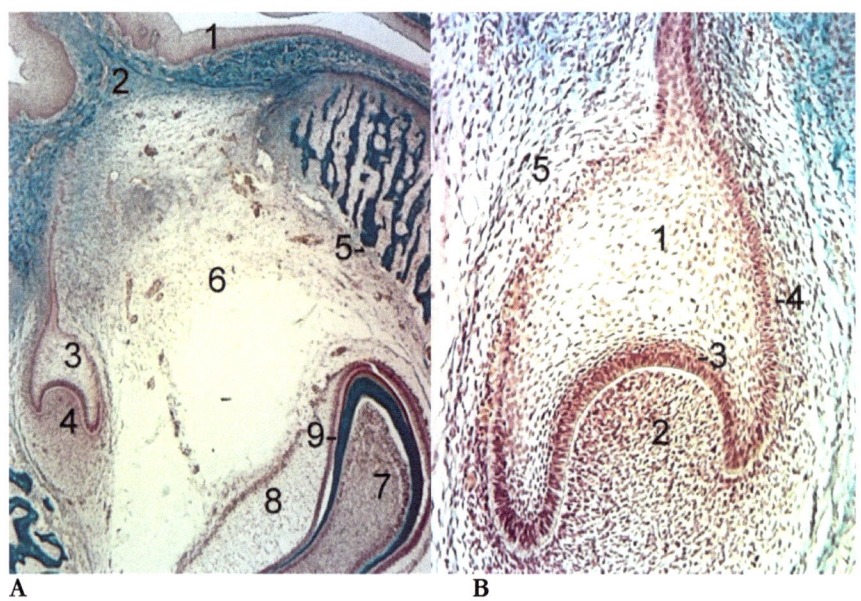

A   B

A Tooth development, sheep embryo, prenatal, Azan, 25x: 1 gum, 2 propria, 3 enamel organ of the permanent tooth, 4 dental papilla, 5 mandibula, 6 alveole, 7 pulp, 8 enamel pulp, 9 enamel and dentin of the deciduous tooth;
B Permanent tooth, 95x: 1 enamel pulp, 2 dental papilla, 3 ameloblastic layer, 4 its outer part, 5 mesodermal follicular sheath.

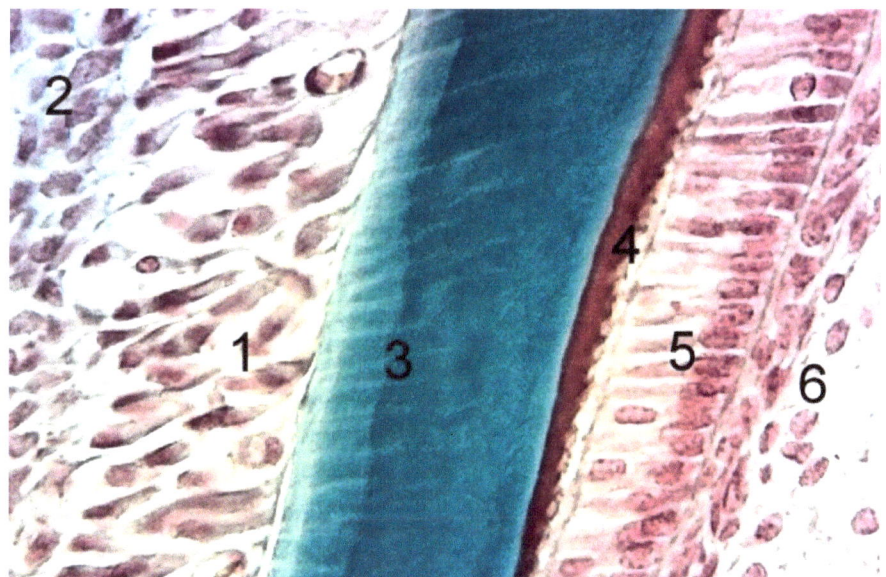

Deciduous tooth, sheep embryo, prenatal, Azan, 375x: 1 ameloblastic layer, 2 ameloblastic pulp, 3 enamel, 4 dentin, 5 odontoblastic layer, 6 dental pulp.

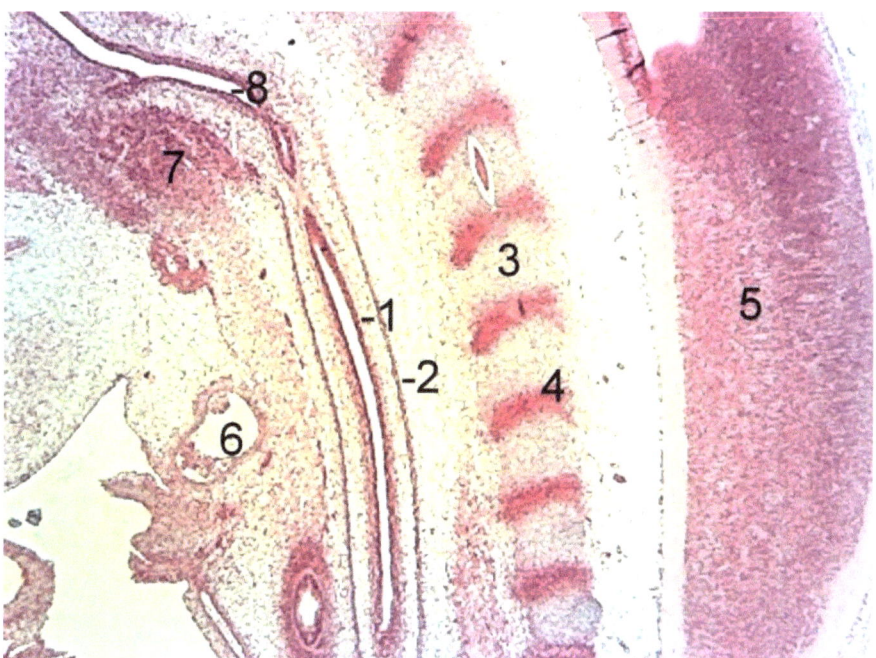

Development of the oesophagus, cat embryo, 25 days, GRA, 25x: 1 oesophagus, 2 its muscle layer, 3 vertebrae, 4 discs, 5 spinal cord, 6 aorta, 7 laryngeal blastem, 8 primitive pharynx.

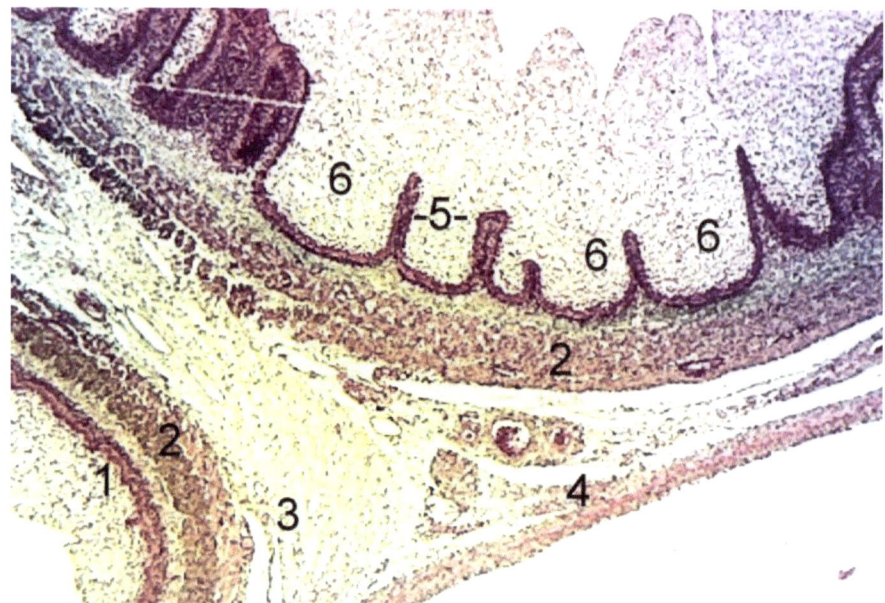

Stomach development, cattle embryo, 30 cm CRL, GRA, 25x: 1 ruminal mucosa, 2 ruminal muscle layer, 3 adventitia, 4 serosa, 5 reticular ridges, 6 reticular cells.

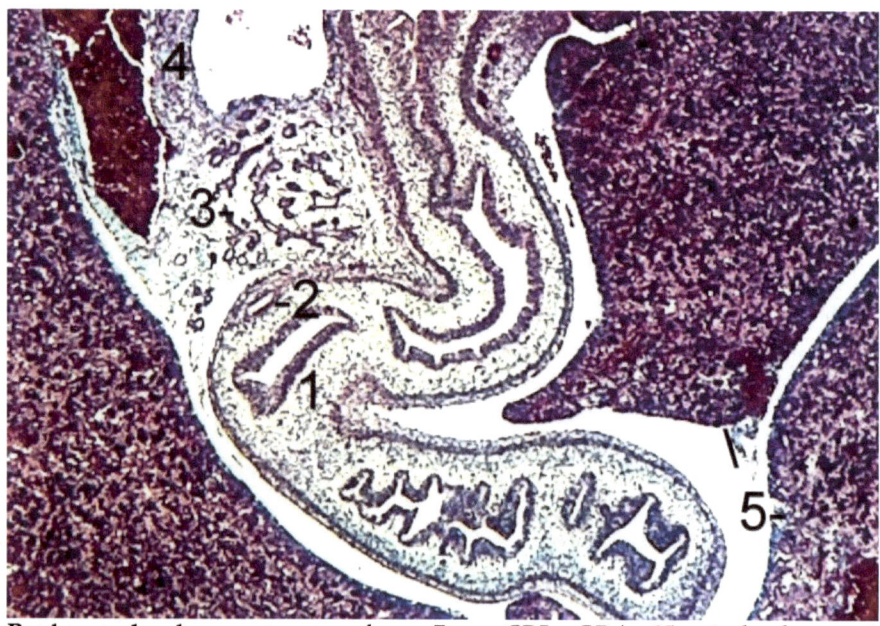

Pankreas development, cat embryo, 7 cm CRL, GRA, 25x: 1 duodenum, 2 pancreatic duct, 3 epithelial sprouts of the primordium, 4 dorsal mesogastrium, 5 liver with haematopoietic spots.

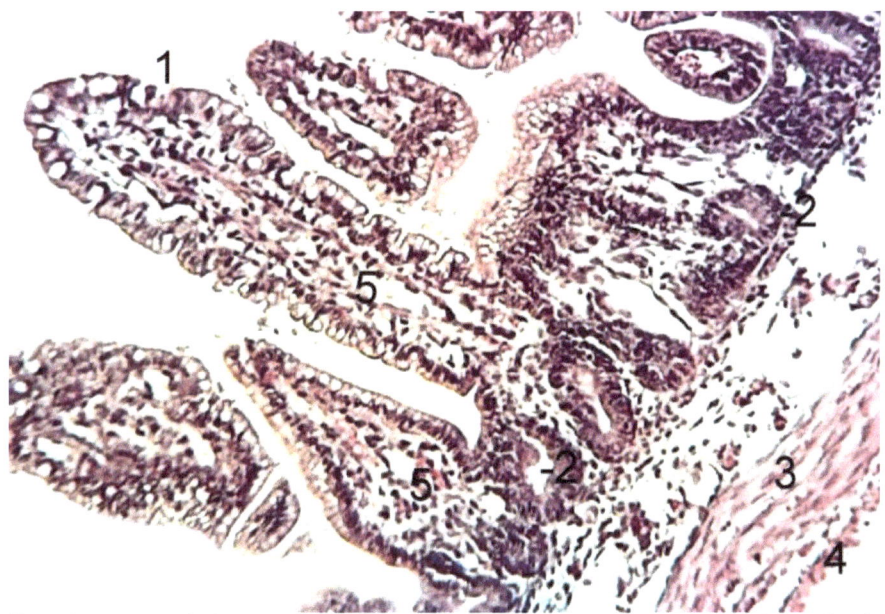

Development of the small intestines, jejunum, cat embryo, 19 cm CRL, GRA, 95x: 1 primitive villi with enterocytes and goblet cells, 2 crypts, 3 muscle layer, 4 serosa.

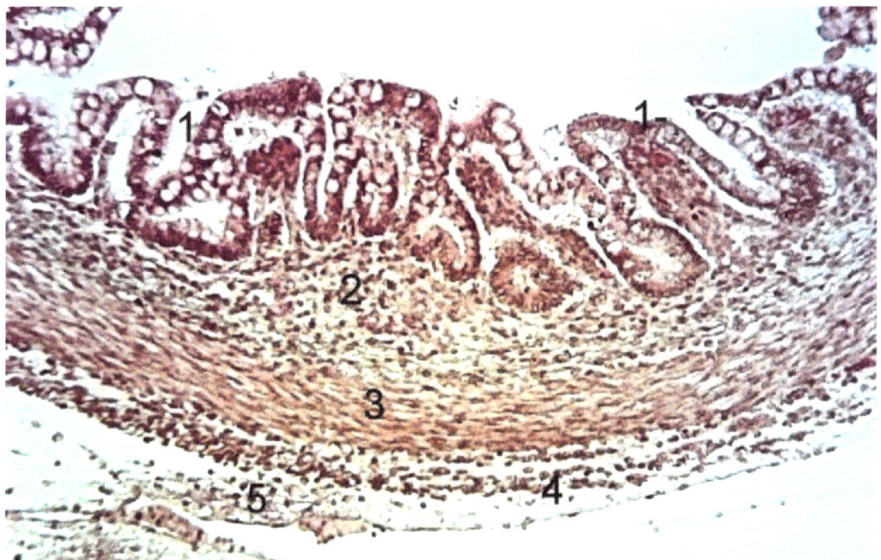

Development of the big intestines, colon, cat embryo, 8cm CRL, GRA, 95x: 1 crypt, 2 follicles, 3 circular muscles, 4 longitudinal muscles, 5 serosa.

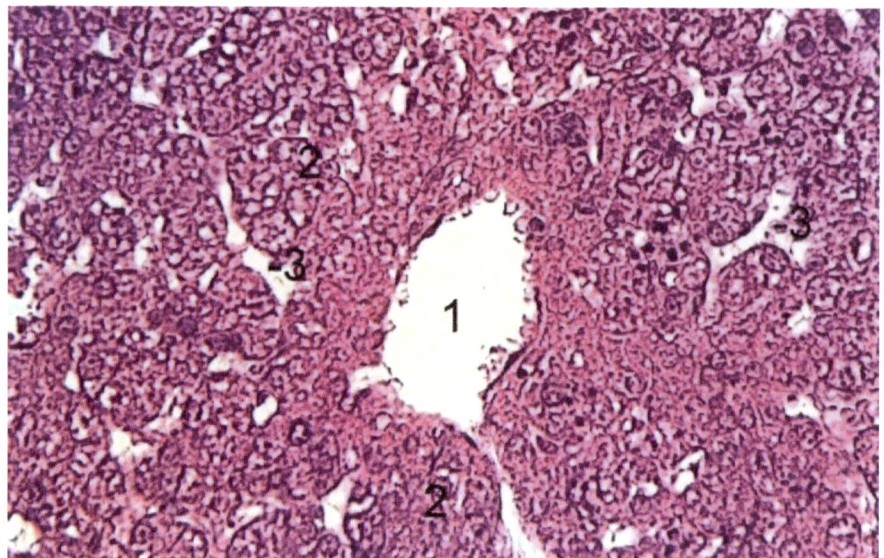
Liver development, dog, newborn, HE, 240x: 1 central vein, 2 lobuli, 3 sinusoids.

9 UROGENITAL APPARATUS

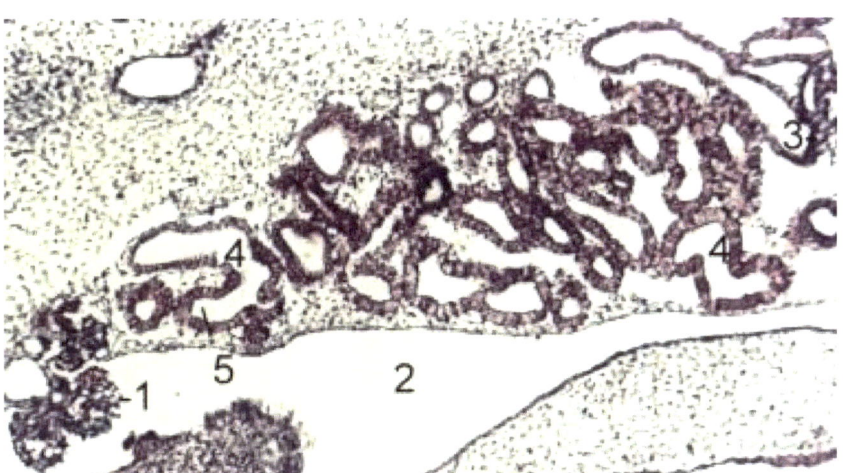

Pro- and mesonephros, cat embryo, 19 days, longitudinal, 240x: 1 outer glomerulus of the pronephros, 2 coelom, 3 inner glomerulus of the mesonephros, 4 tubuli, 5 Wolffian duct.

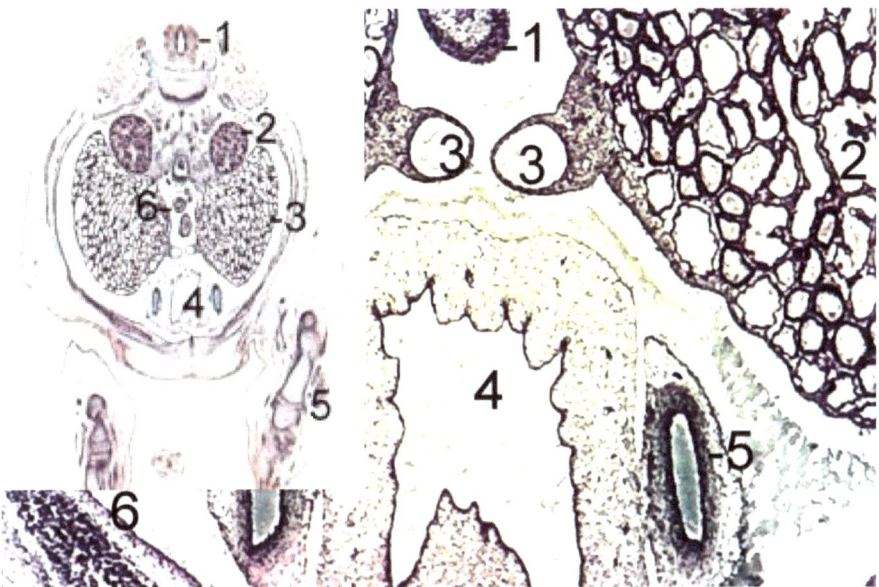

Mesonephros, pig embryo, 3,7 cm CRL, cross, GRA, 25x: 1 colon, 2 mesonephros, 3 Wolffian duct, 4 urogenital sinus, 5 umbilical arteries, 6 body wall. Overview: 1 spinal cord, 2 metanephros, 3 mesonephros, 4 urogenital sinus, 5 limb, 6 colon.

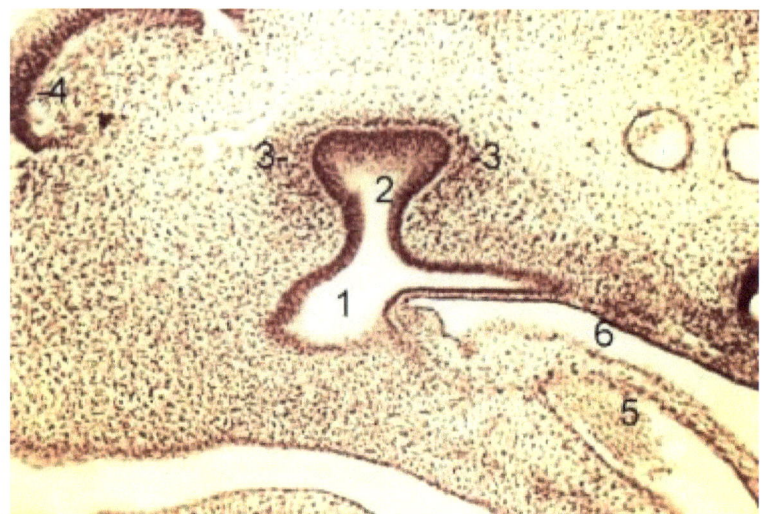

Metanephros (permanent kidney), cat embryo, 14 days, HE, 95x: 1 Wolffian duct, 2 ureteric bud, 3 metanephrogenic blastema, 4 dermatomyotom, 5 subcardinal vein, 6 coelom.

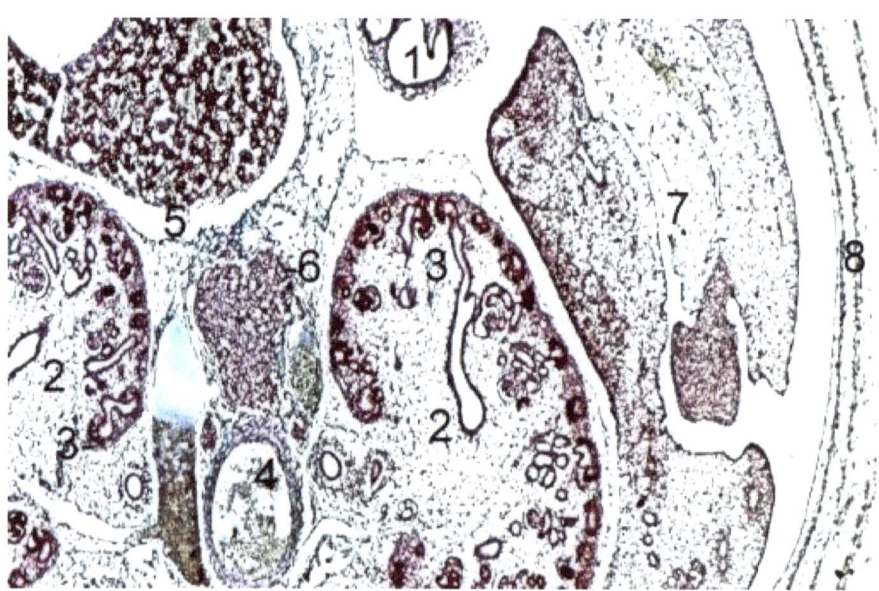

Kidney, cat embryo, 28 Tage, horizontal, GRA, 25x: 1 Wolffian duct, 2 metanephros, 3 dichotome ureteric sprouts induce nephric corpuscles, 4 aorta, 5 liver, 6 suprarenal, 7 urogenital fold, 8 body wall.

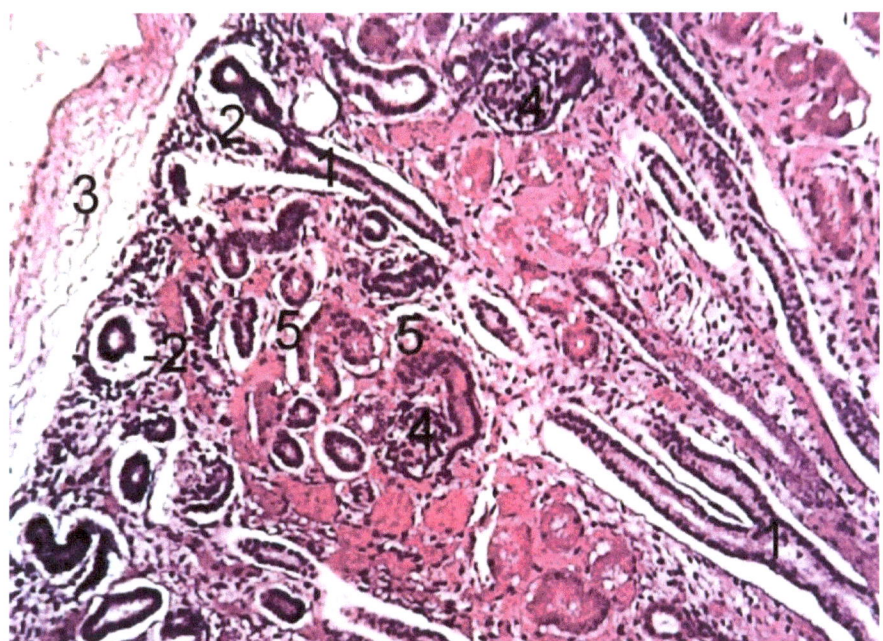

Kidney, cat embryo, last trimester, HE, 95x: 1 ureteric sprouts, 2 nephric corpuscles, 3 capsule, 4 developing glomeruli, 5 developing tubules.

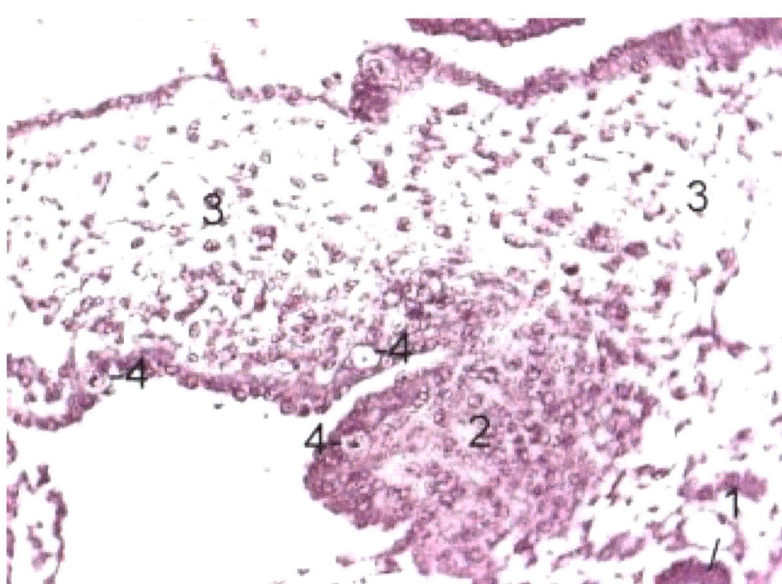

Genital ridge, cat embryo, 19 days, cross, 240x: 1 mesonephros, 2 genital ridge, 3 mesentery, 4 primordial germ cells.

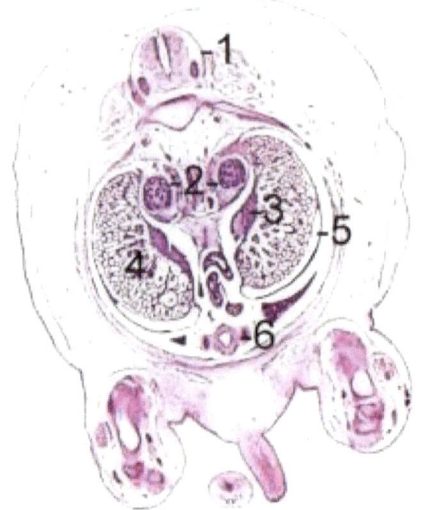

Genital ridge, sheep embryo, 3,5 cm CRL, cross section, GRA, 15x: 1 spinal cord, 2 metanephros, 3 gential ridge, 4 mesonephros, 5 Wolffian duct, 6 urogenital sinus.

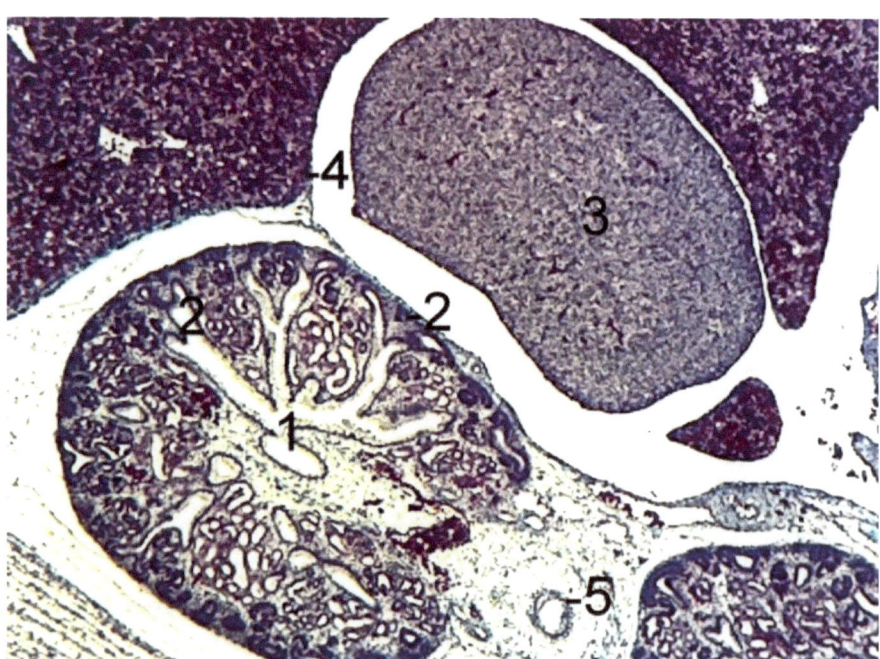

Indifferent gonad, cat embryo, 7 cm CRL, GRA, 25x: 1 kidney, 2 ureteric sprouts with nephric corpuscles and nephric tubules, 3 gonade, 4 liver, 5 ureter.

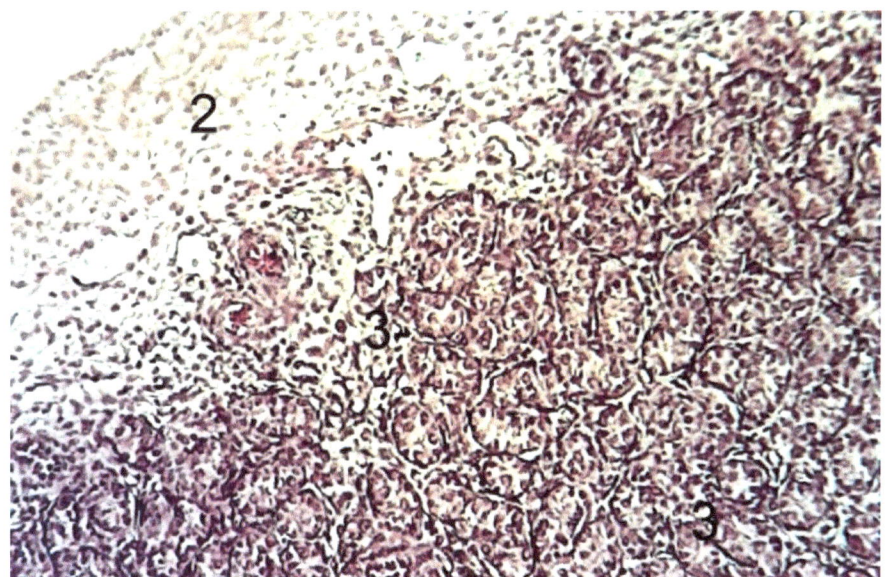

Testicular development, sheep embryo, 20 cm CRL, GRA, 240x: 2 capsule, 3 primitive testicular tubules.

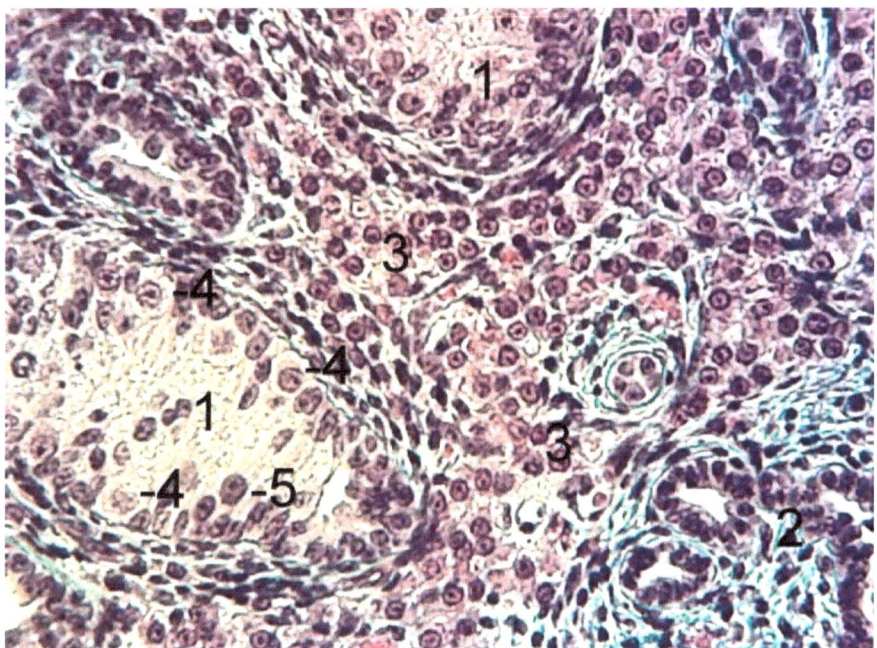

Testis, cat, prenatal, GRA, 240x: 1 primitive testicular tubules, 2 mesonephric tubules, 3 intermediate cells, 4 gonocyten, 5 sertoli cells.

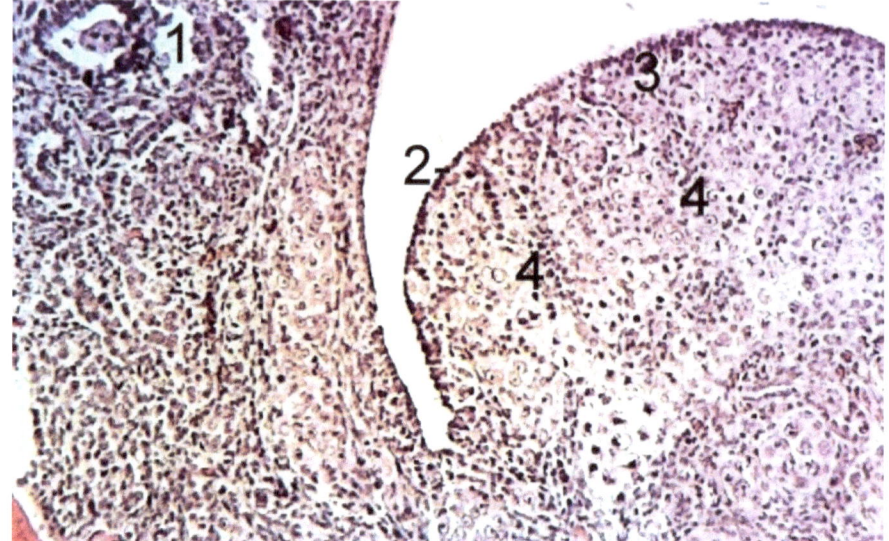

Ovarial development, cat, prenatal, GRA, 95x: 1 mesonephros, 2 germinal epithelium, 3 epithelial strands, 4 intermediate cells.

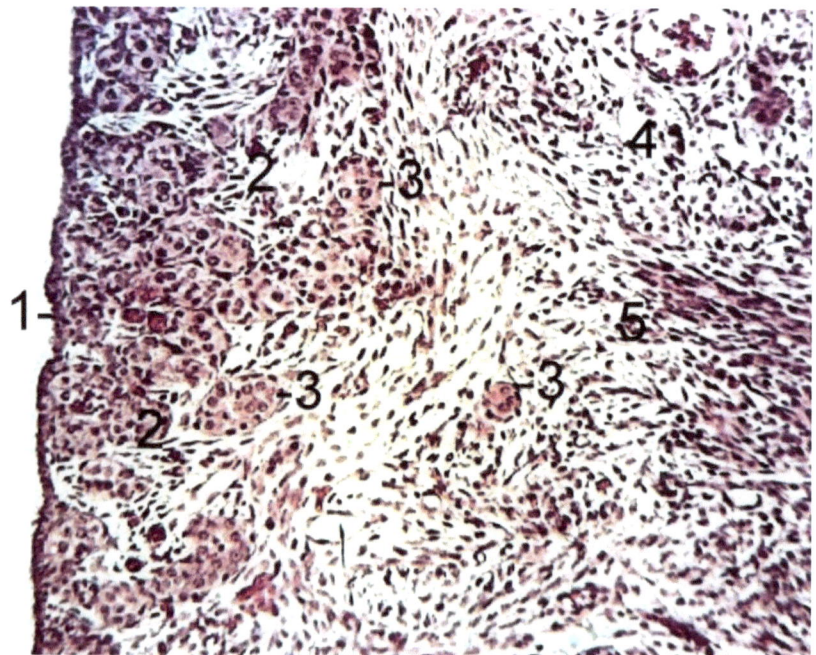

Ovary, dog, newborn, GRA, 95x: 1 germinal epithelium, 2 epithelial strands, 3 isolated clusters, 4 vessels of the medulla, 5 intermediate cells.

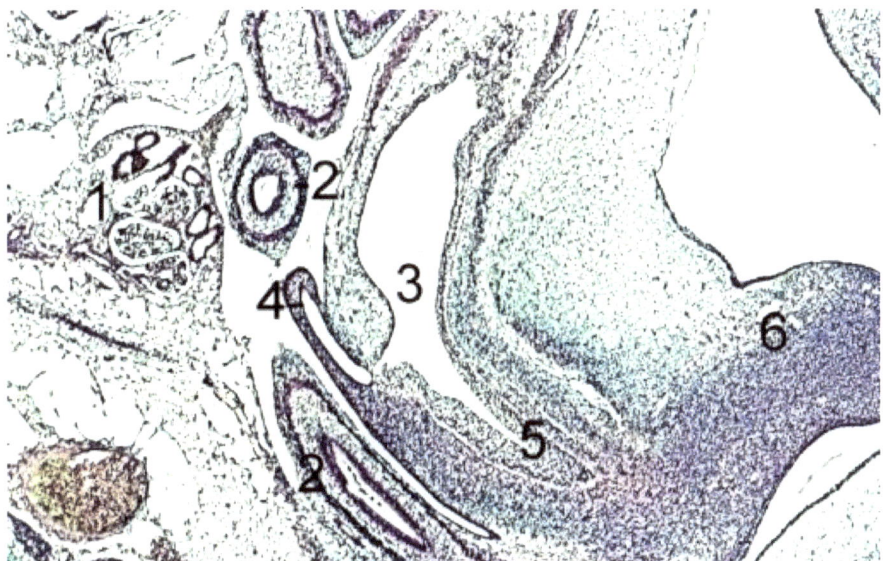
Urogenital sinus, cat embryo, 25 days, GRA, 25x: 1 mesonephric remnants, 2 rectum, 3 urogenital sinus, 4 Wolffian duct, 5 urachus, 6 phallus.

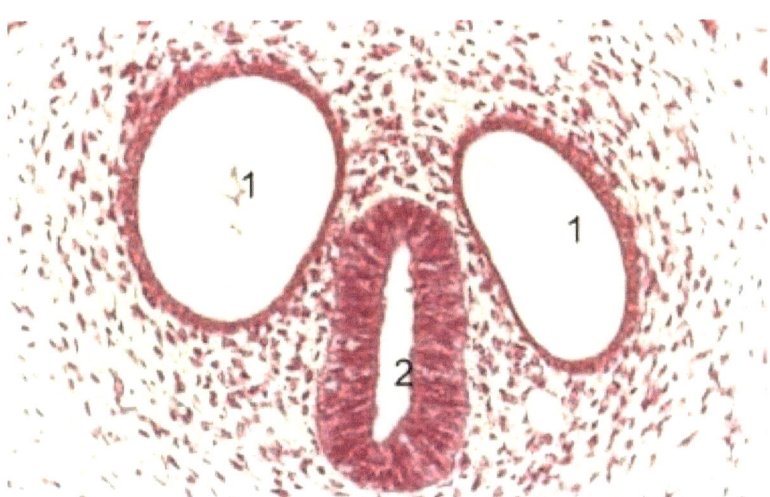
Development of the uterus, sheep embryo, 3,5 cm CRL, HE, 240x: 1 Wolffian ducts, 2 fused Mullerian ducts as primordium of the uterus body.

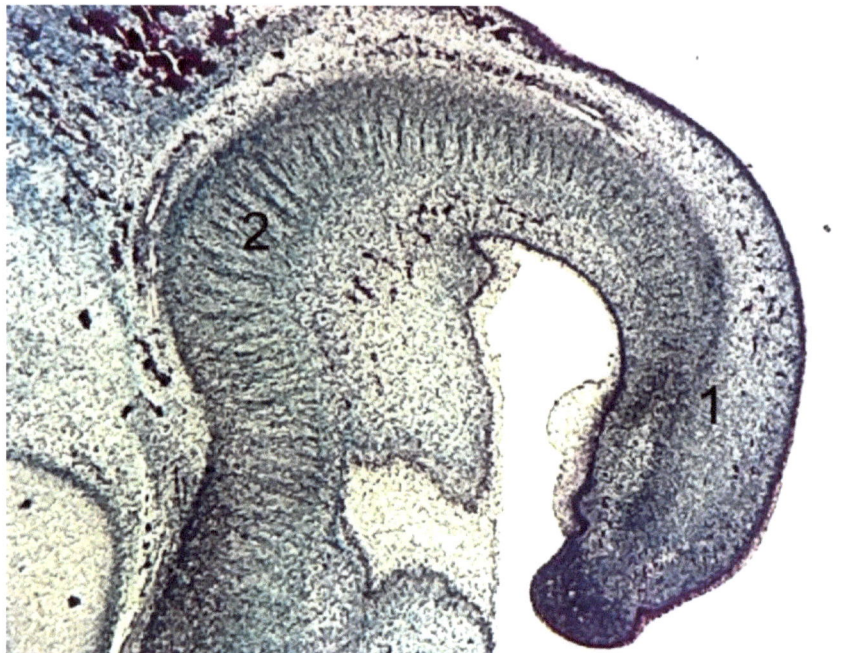

Development of the penis, cat embryo, 7 cm CRL, GRA, 25x: 1 primordium of the spongiose body, 2 primordium of the cavernose body.

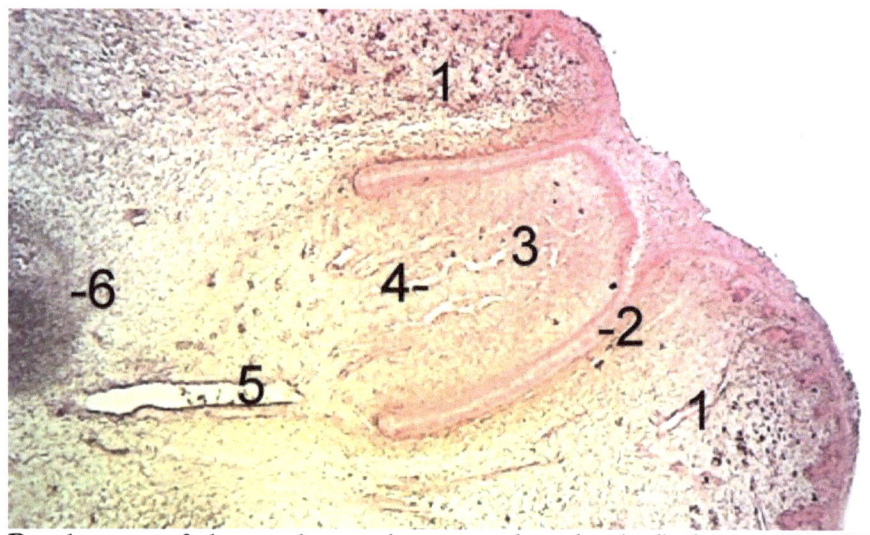

Development of glans and preputium, cat embryo, longitudinal, 8 cm CRL, HE, 25x: 1 preputial skin, 2 glandar lamella, 3 glans, 4 cavernose body, 5 urethra, 6 primordium of the penile bone.

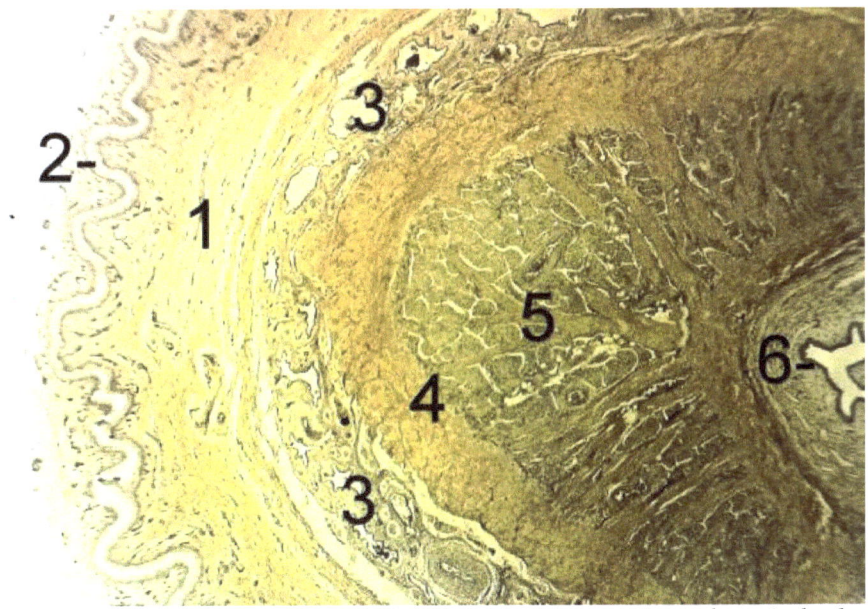

Penis differentiation, horse, prenatal, cross, van Gieson, 15x: 1 glans, 2 glandar lamella, 3 cavernose body, 4 its capsule 5 trabecles and cavernae, 6 urethra.

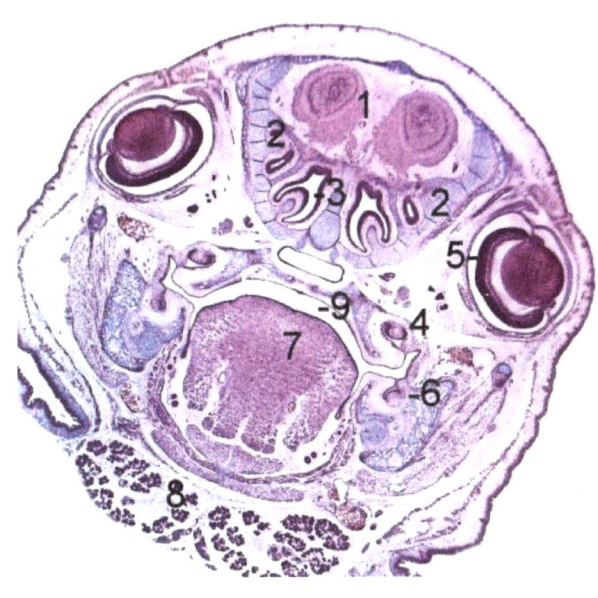

Overview of the next page picture, below: head rat, prenatal, cross section, GRA, 15x: 1 olfactory bulb, 2 ethmoid, 3 nasal fundus, 4 maxillary tooth, 5 eye, 6 mandi-bulary tooth, 7 tongue, 8 neck muscles, 9 oral cavity.

10 NERVOUS SYSTEM

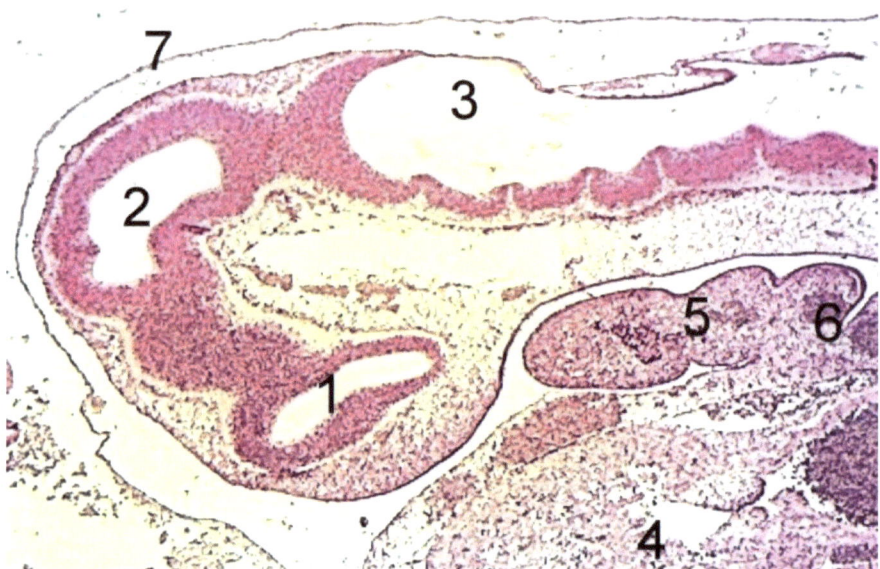

Brain development, cattle embryo, 1 cm CRL, längs, HE, 25x: 1 prosencephalon, 2 mesencephalon, 3 rhombencephalon, 4 heart, 5 first-, 6 second pharyngeal arch, 7 amnion.

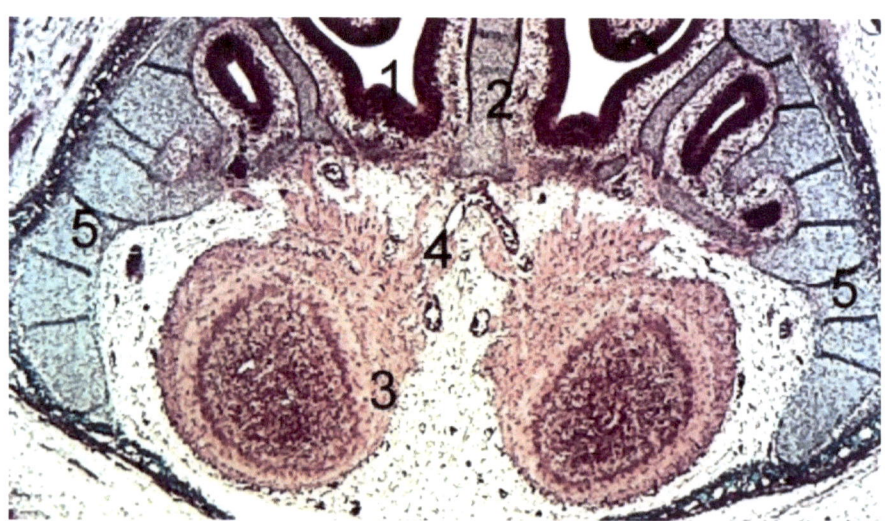

Olfactory bulb, head, rat embryo, cross, 25x: 1 nasal cavity, 2 nasal septum, 3 olfactory bulb, 4 olfactory nerve, 5 primordium of the ethmoid.

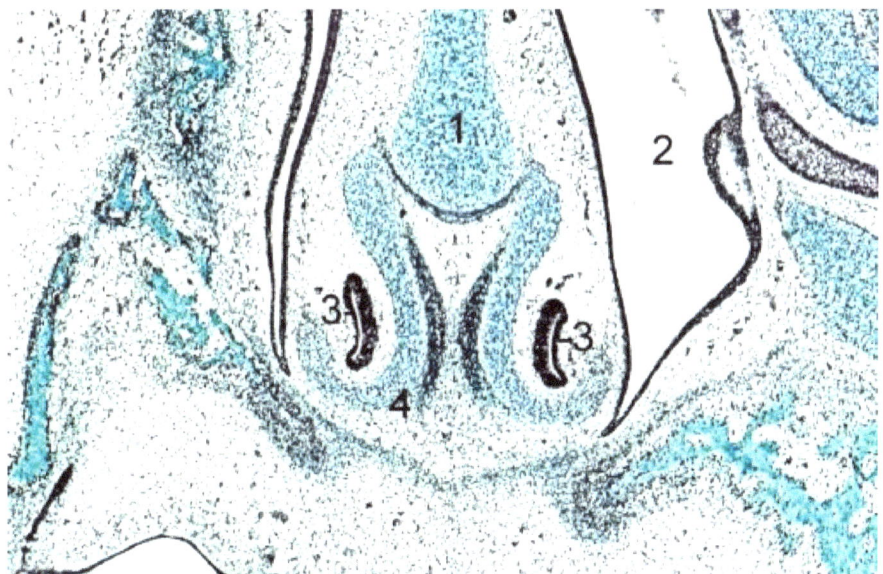

Vomeronasal organ, cat embryo, 34 days, head, cross, GRA, 25x: 1 nasal septum, 2 nasal cavity, 3 primordium of the vomeronasal organ, 4 vomeral cartilage.

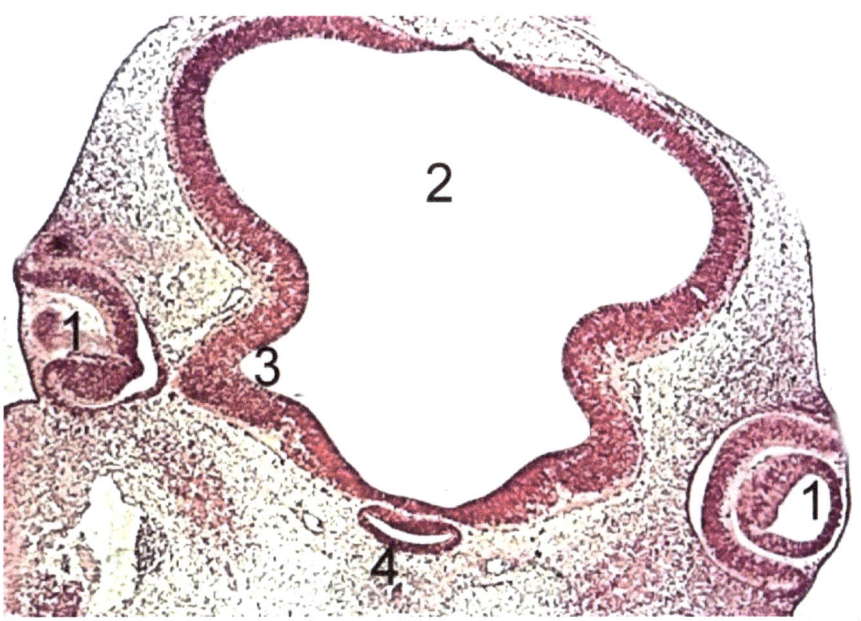

Development of the eye, sheep embryo, 2,8 cm CRL, cross, GRA, 25x: 1 optic cup, 2 midbrain vesicle, 3 optic recess of the diencephalic vesicle, 4 Rathke's pouch.

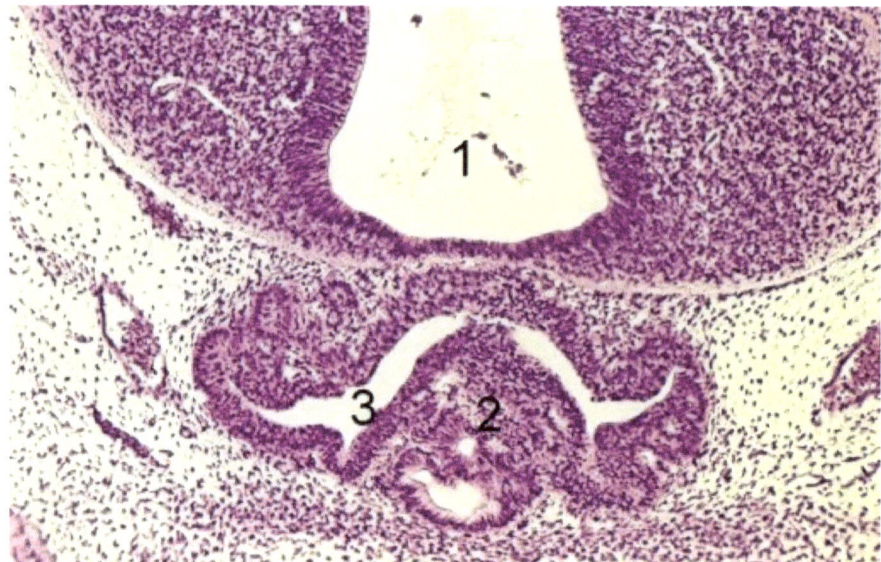

Development of the hypophysis, sheep embryo, 2,9 cm CRL, cross, HE, 25x: 1 diencephalic vesicle, 2 middle part, 3 lateral part of the adenohypophysis.

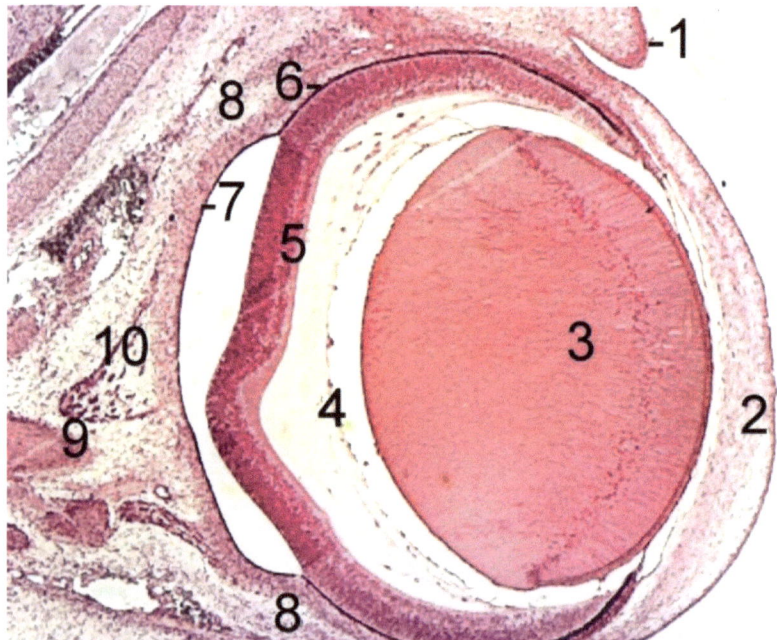

Development of the optic bulb, sheep embryo, 3,5 cm CRL, cross, HE, 25x: 1 eyelid, 2 cornea, 3 lens, 4 vitreous body, 5 retina, 6 pigment layer, 7 chorioid primordium, 8 primordium of the sclera, 9 optic nerve, 10 eye muscles.

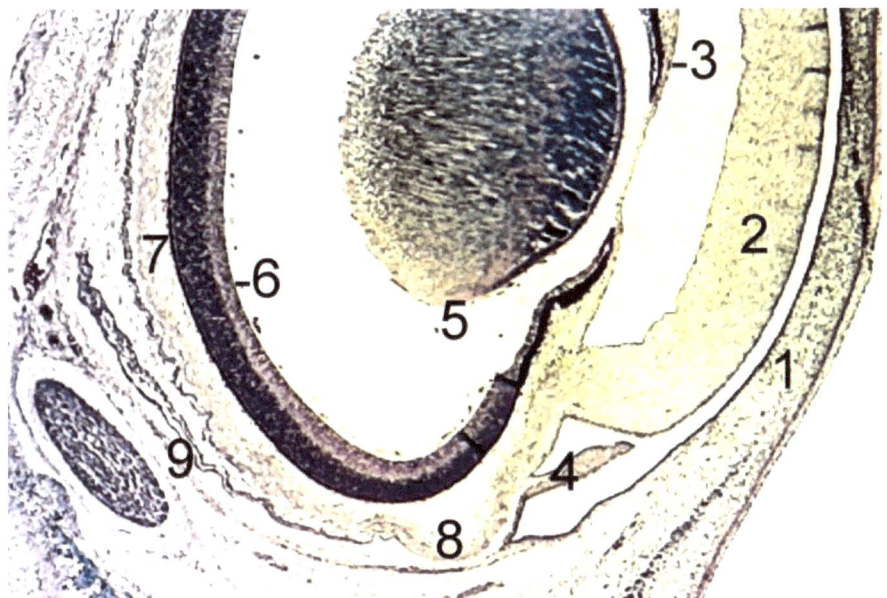

Differentiation of the eye, pig embryo, 6 cm CRL, quer, GRA, 25x: 1 lid, 2 cornea, 3 iris, 4 third eye lid, 5 lens and ciliary body, 6 retina, 7 chorioidea, 8 sclera, 9 eye muscles and optiv nerve.

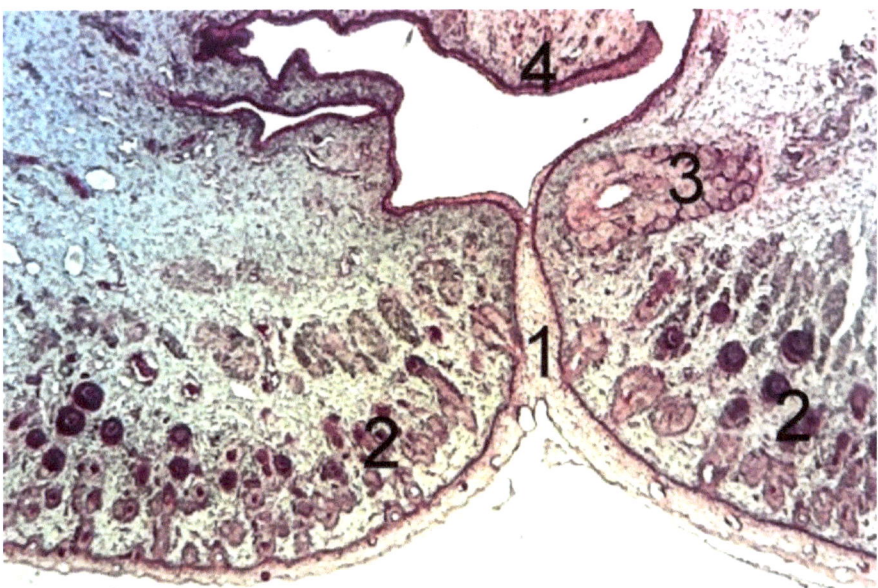

Development of the lid, sheep embryo, 30 cm CRL, cross, GRA, 25x: 1 synechia of the lid, 2 hair and gland primordia, 3 primordium of Meiboms gland, 4 third eye lid.

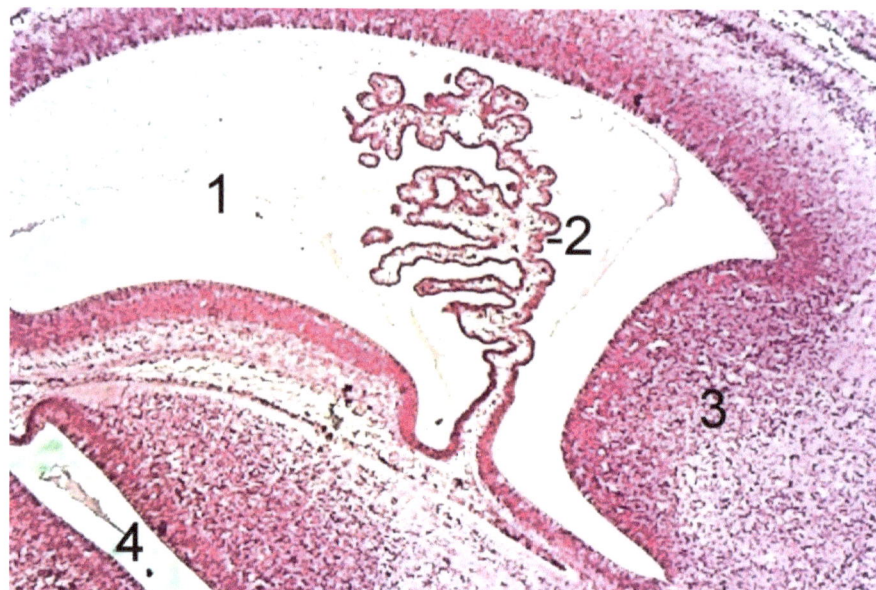

Development of the cerebrum, sheep embryo, 3,5 cm CRL, HE, 25x: 1 ventricle, 2 chorioid plexus, 3 caudate nucleus, 4 plexus of the third ventricle.

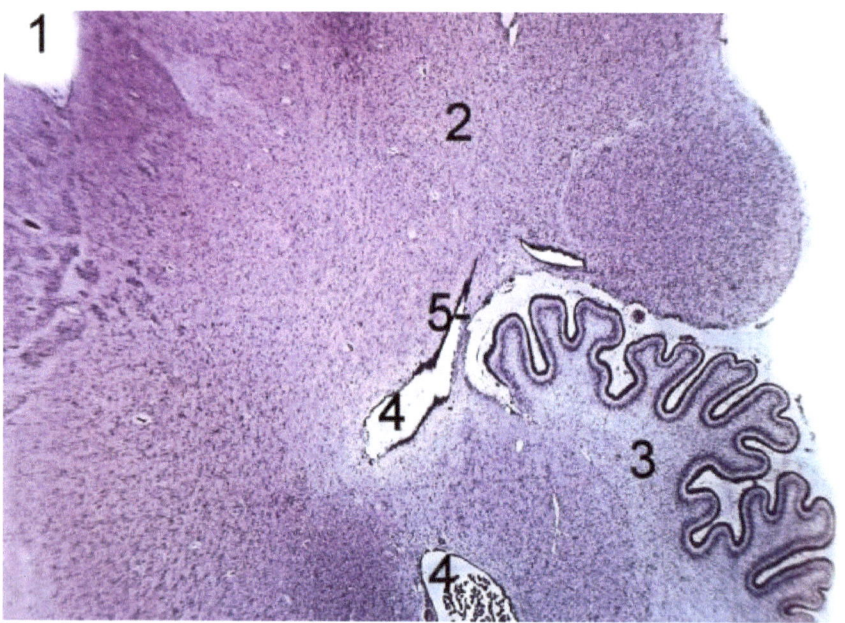

Development of the cerebellum, dog embryo, prenatal, GRA, 25x: 1 ventricle, 2 cerebrum, 3 cerebellum, 4 aqueduct and plexus, 5 anterior velum.

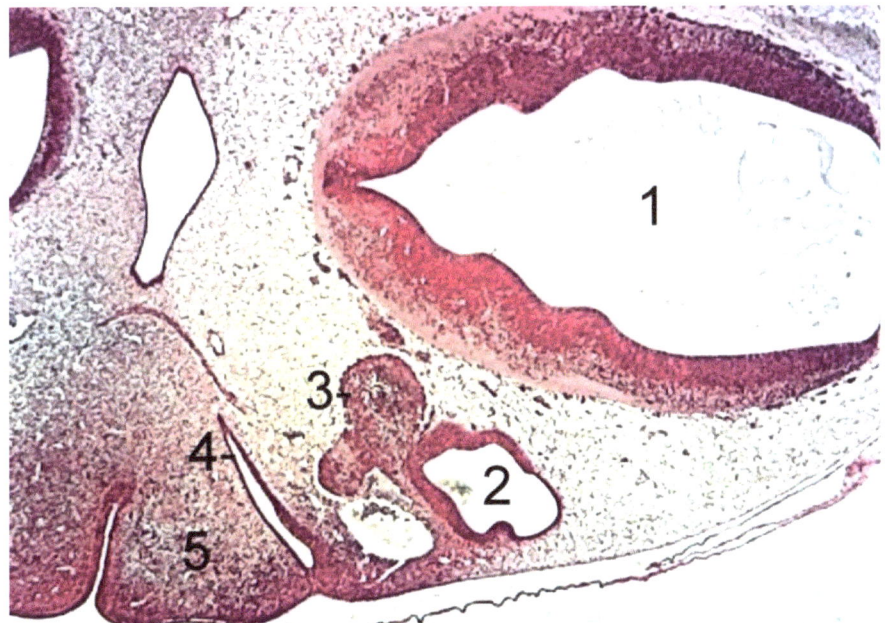

Otic vesicle, sheep embryo, 2,8 CRL, GRA, 25x: 1 rhombencephalon, 2 otic vesicle, 3 vestibulocochlear ganglion, 4 first pharyngeal cleft, 5 first pharyngeal arch.

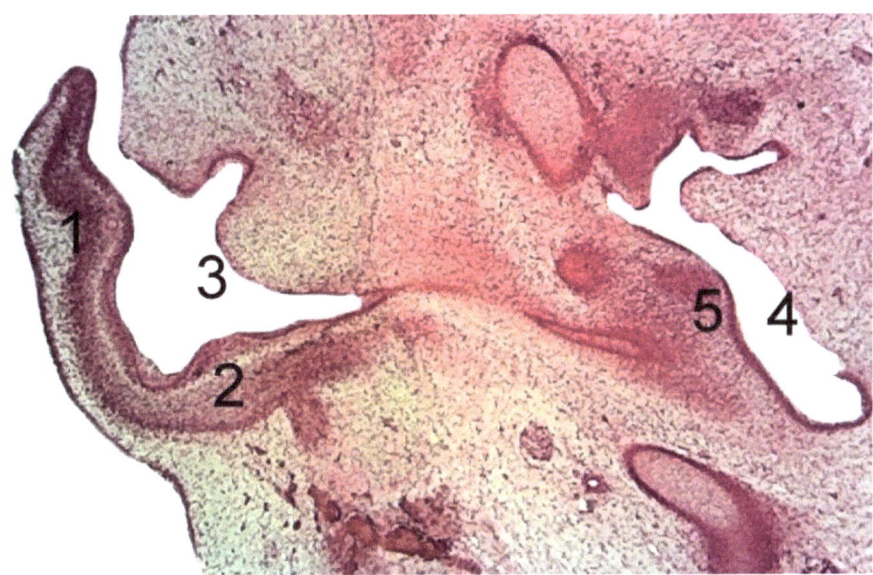

Development of the ear, sheep embryo, 3,5 cm CRL, GRA, 25x: 1 external ear, 2 its cartilage, 3 external otic meatus, 4 endolymphatic part, 5 tympanic membran.

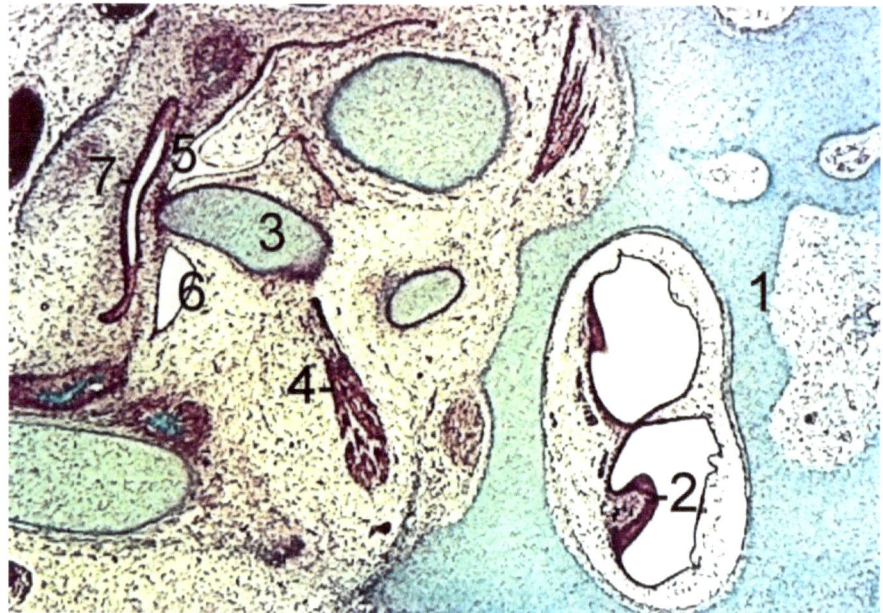

Development of the inner ear, car embryo, 26 days, GRA, 25x: 1 petrosal cartilage, 2 macula primordium of the labyrinth ampulla, 3 malleus cartilage, 4 blastema of the tensor tympani muscle, 5 tympanic membrane, 6 epitympanic cavity, 7 external meatus.

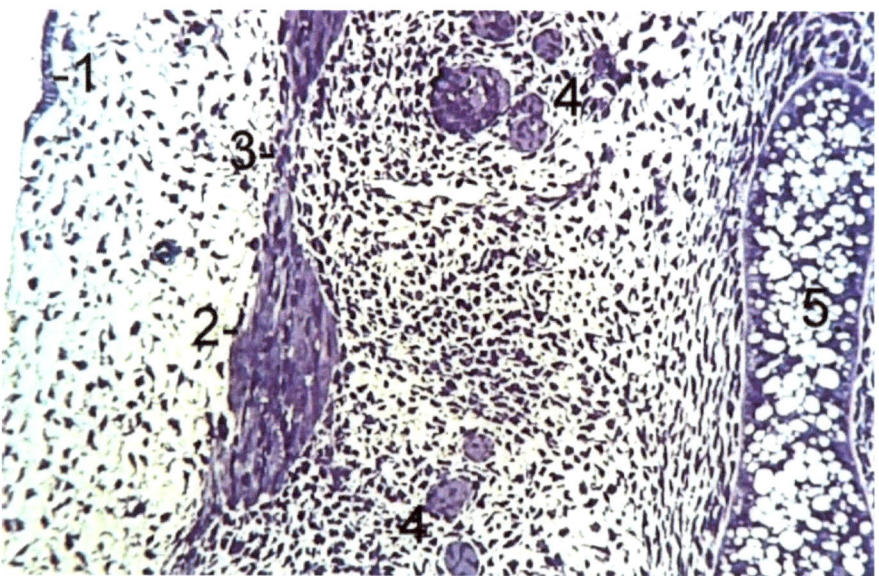

Development of the sympathic cord, duck embryo, 5 days, Richardson, 95x: 1 ectoderm, 2 ganglia primordia, 3 interganglionar ramus, 4 splanchnic nerves, 5 notochord.

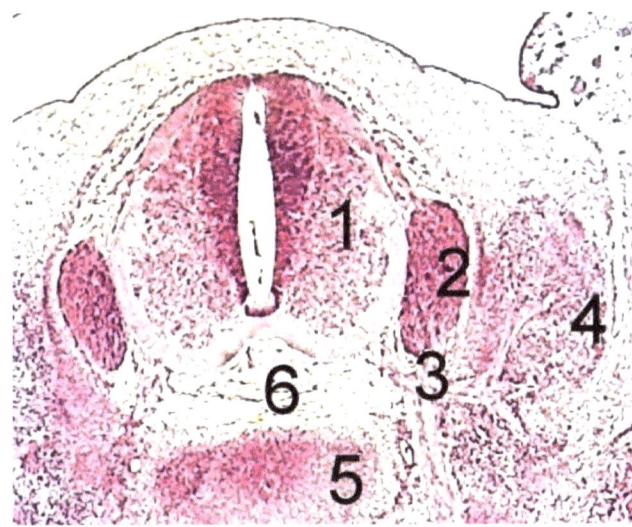

Spinal cord and spinal nerves, sheep embryo, 2 cm CRL, HE, 25x: 1 spinal cord, 2 spinal-ganglion, 3 spinal nerve, 4 epimer, 5 vertebral body.

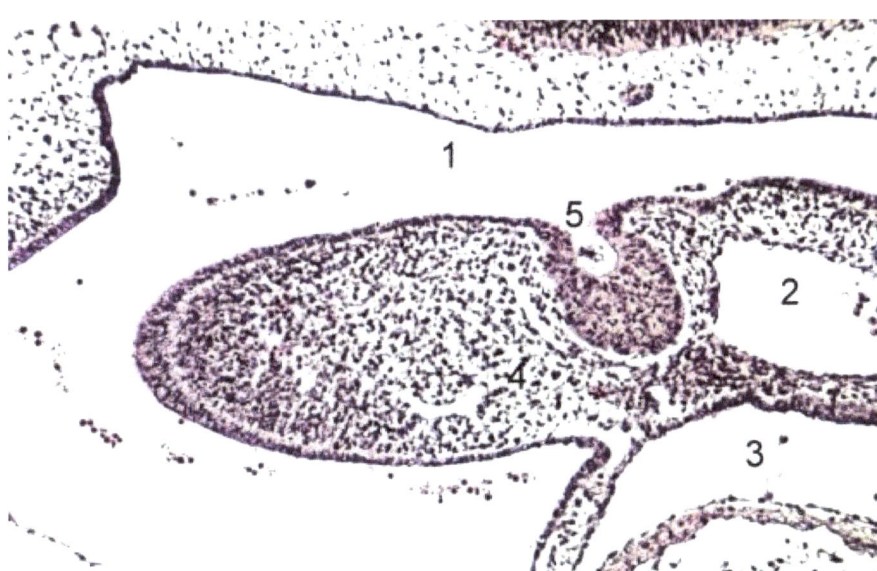

Thyroid development, cat embryo, 17 days, longitudinal, HE, 95x: 1 primitive pharynx, 2 pharyngeal artery, 3 pericardial cavity, 4 first pharyngeal arch, 5 thyroid placode.

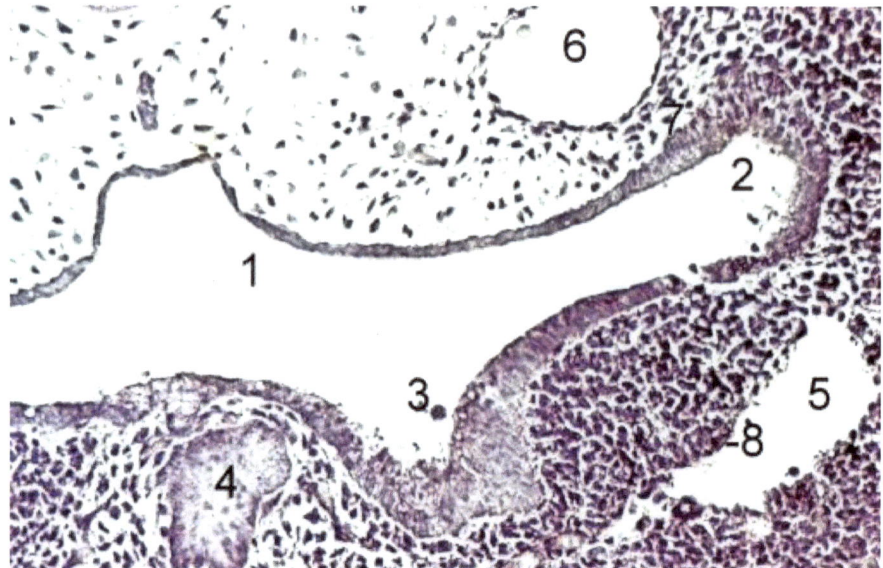

Derivatives of the pharyngeal pouches, horse embryo, 21 days, cross, GRA, 240x: 1 primitive pharynx, 2 dorsal recess of the third pouch with the primordium of the parathyroid, 3 ventral recess of the third pouch, 4 thyroid vesicle, 5 third pharyngeal artery, 6 dorsal aorta, 8 thymic primordium.

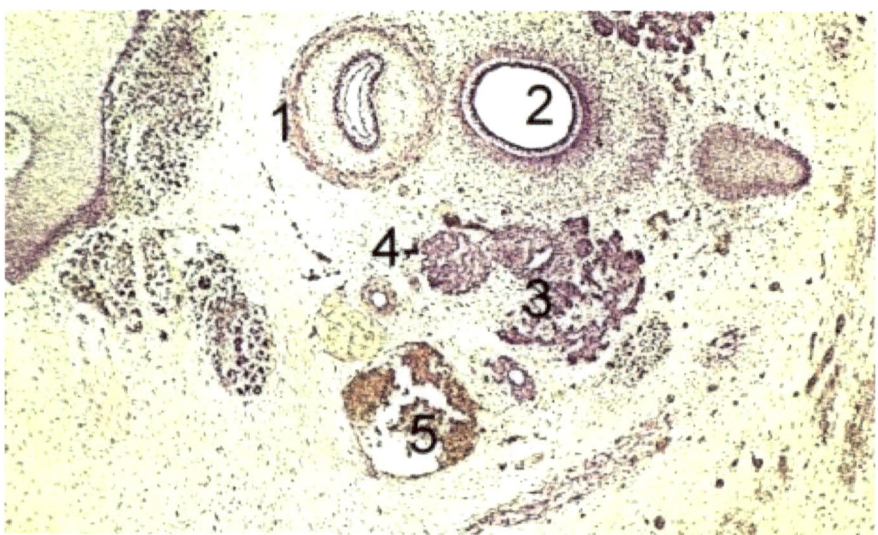

Topogenesis of the thyroid gland, sheep embryo, 3 cm CRL, GRA, 25x: 1 oesophagus, 2 trachea, 3 thyroid, 4 third parathyroid, 5 carotid.

Pictures of Veterinary Embryology

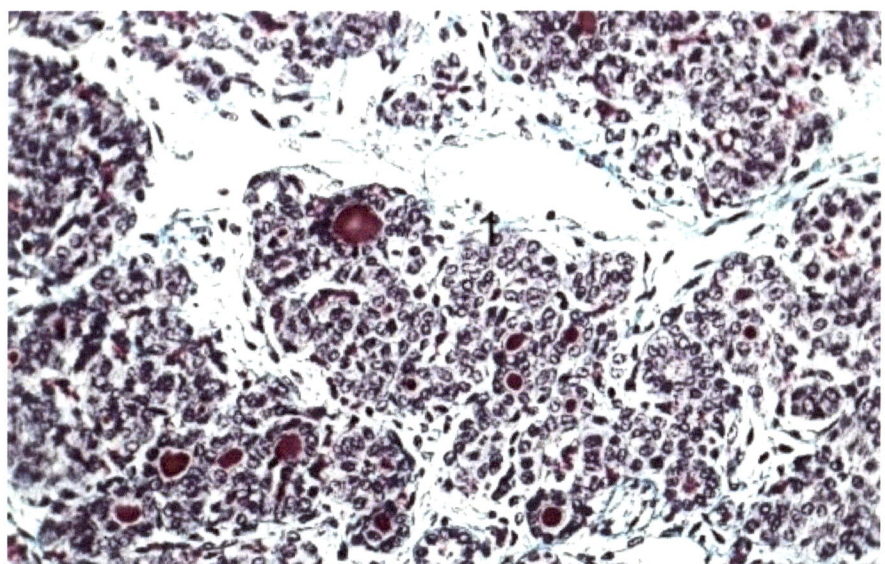

Histogenesis of the thyroid, cattle embryo, 22cm CRL, GRA, 240x: 1 first follicles with colloid (red).

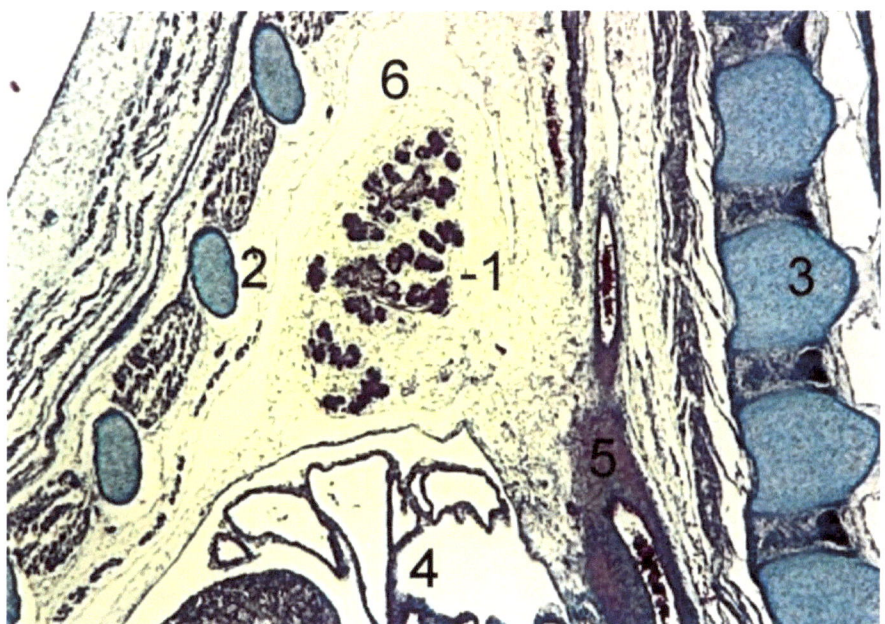

Differentiation of the thymus, cat embryo, 32 days, long., GRA, 25x: 1 primitive lobules, 2 rip cartilages, 3 vertebrae, 4 atrium, 5 aorta, 6 cupula pleurae.

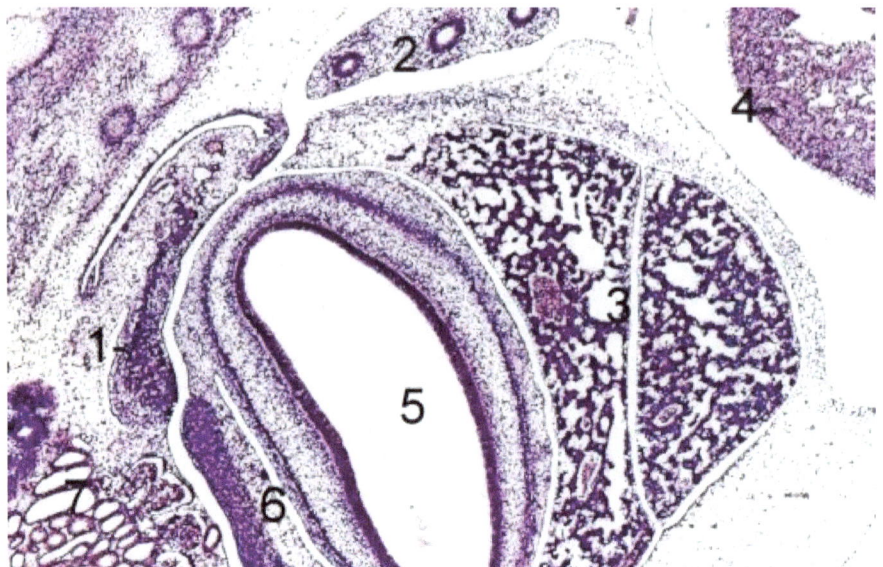

Development of the supra renal, cat embryo, 25 days, long, GRA, 25x: 1 suprarenal blastem, 2 lung, 3 liver, 4 heart, 5 stomach, 6 spleen.

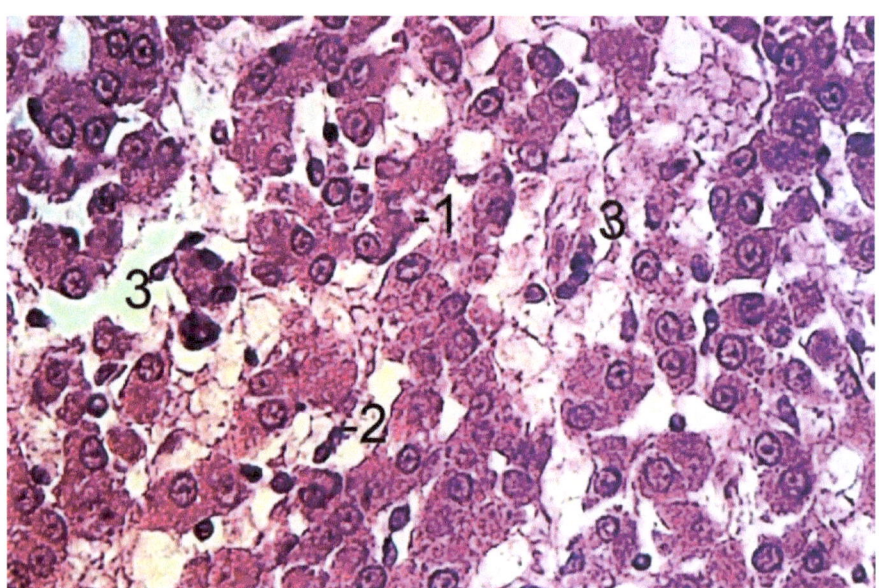

Suprarenal differentiation, cat embryo, 28 days, cross, HE, 375x: 1 epithelial strands, 2 mesenchyme, 3 plexus.

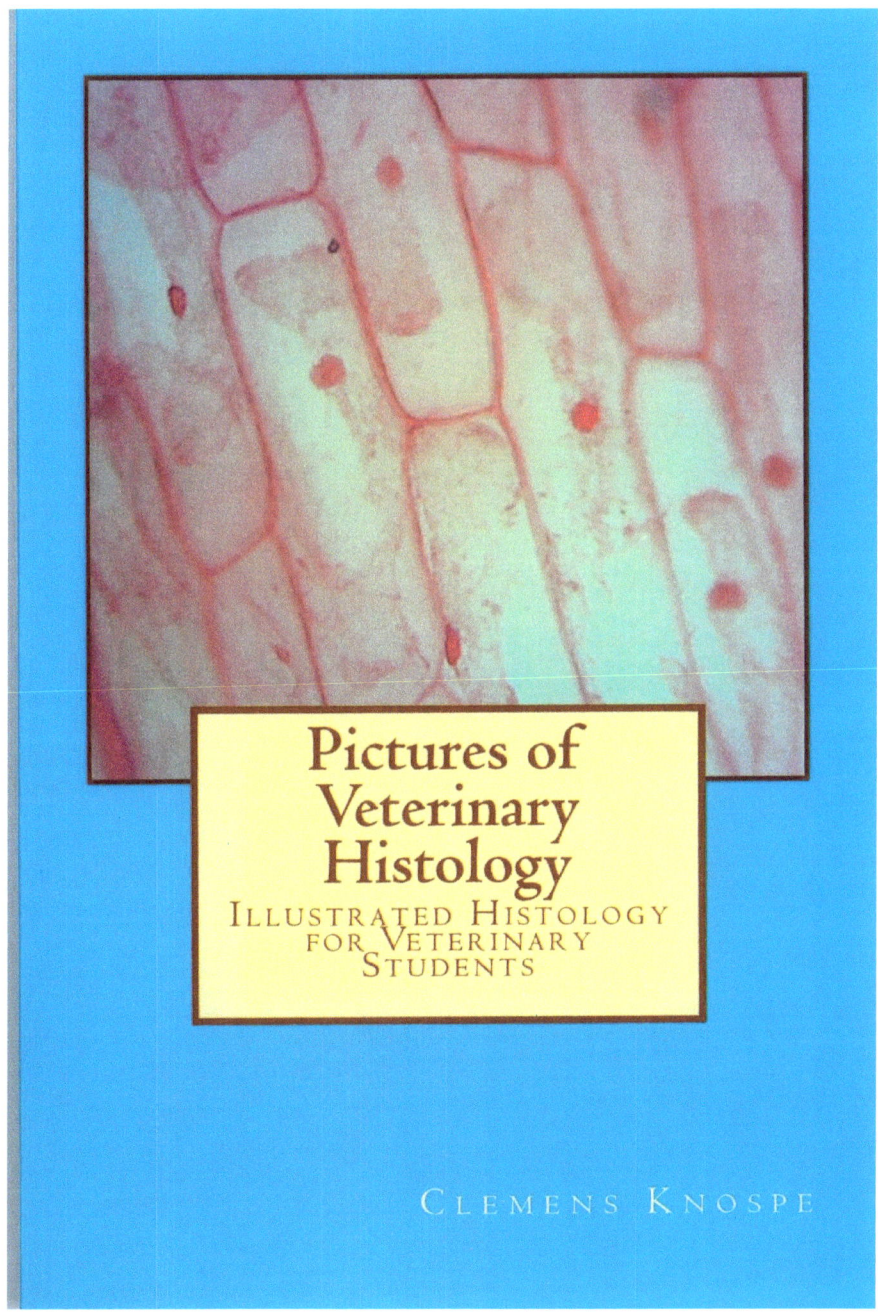

CLEMENS KNOSPE

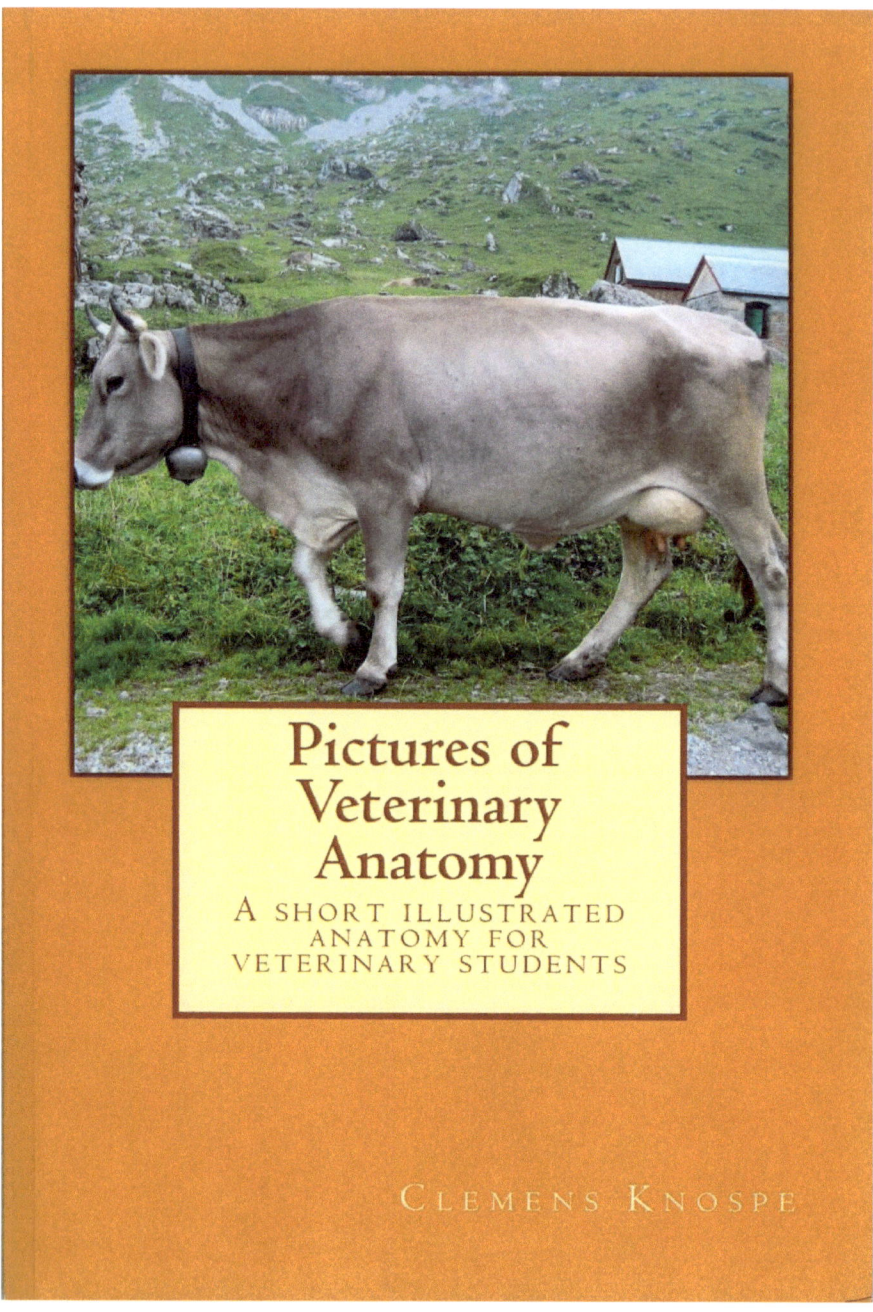

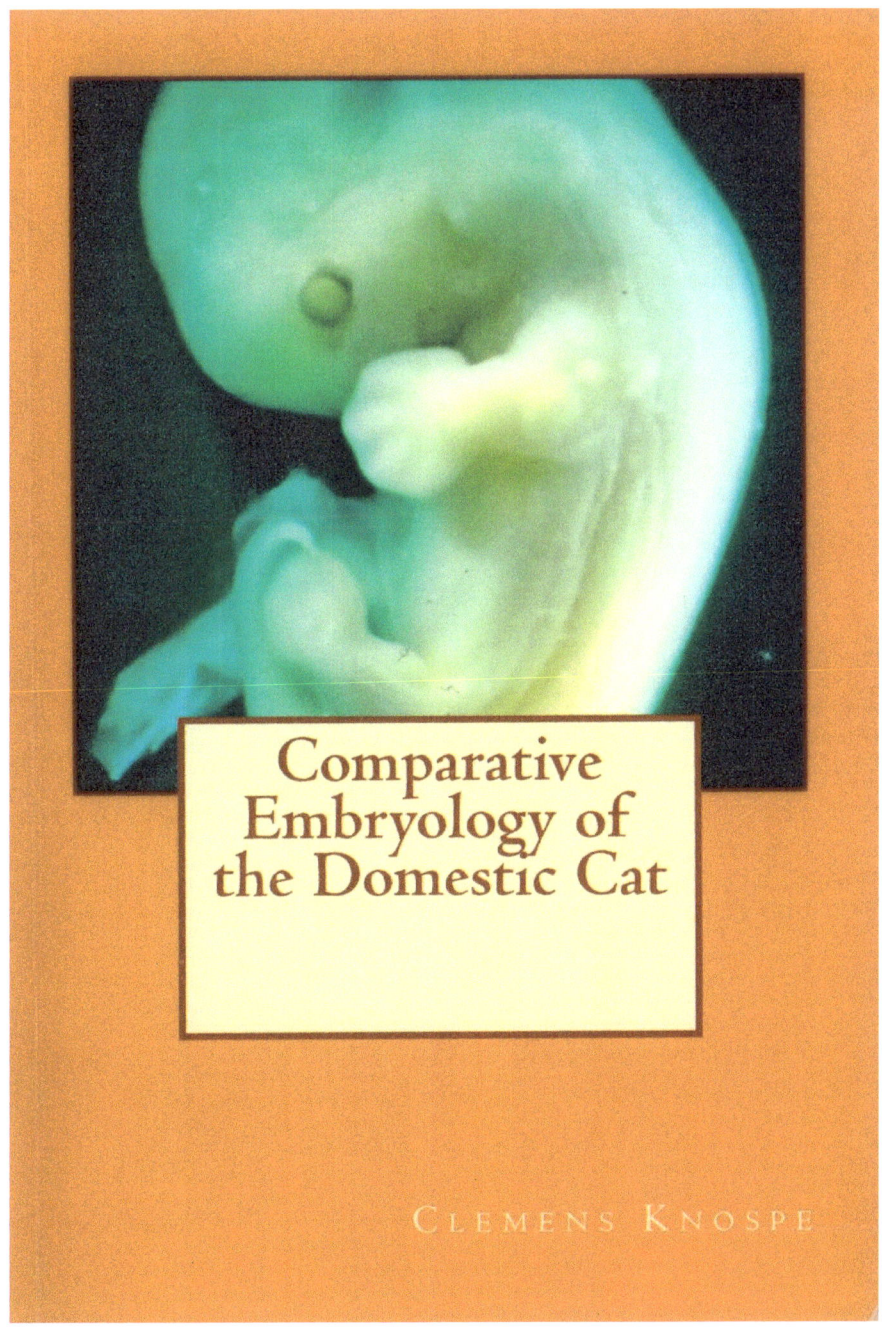

Dr. Clemens Knospe is Professor for Veterinary-Anatomy,
-Histology and -Embryology at the LMU Munich.

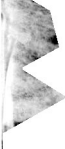

www.ingramcontent.com/pod-product-compliance
Lightning Source LLC
Chambersburg PA
CBHW040807200526
45159CB00022B/47